🎁 **Join Our Community on Facebook for Exclusive Content!**

Scan the QR Code Below 🎁

Disclaimer

The information provided in this book is intended for educational and informational purposes only. It is not a substitute for professional medical advice, diagnosis, or treatment. Always seek the advice of your physician or other qualified healthcare provider before starting any new fitness program or making any changes to an existing one. The author and publisher of this book are not responsible for any injury or health problems that may result from the use of the information in this book.

- A Bonus with Relaxation Breathing Techniques and a Nutritional Guide you can download.
  It helps you follow your exercises easily.

- A special way to text me if you have questions or just want to say hi!

  Don't like texting? No problem! Email me anytime at **avfitness99coaching@gmail.com.**

  I'm here to help you with your fitness!

Contents

CHAIR EXERCISES FOR SENIORS STRETCHING POSES

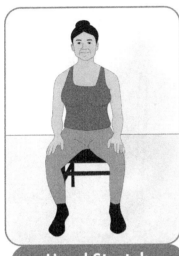

Hand Stretch Pose

Pag 08

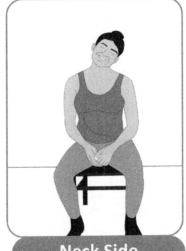

Neck Side to Side

Pag 10

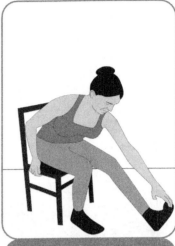

Chair Calf Stretch

Pag 12

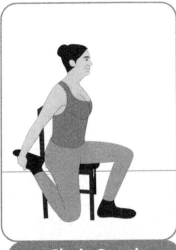

Chair Quad Stretch

Pag 14

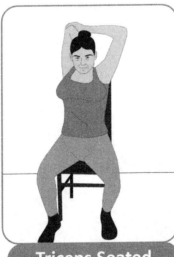

Triceps Seated Stretch

Pag 16

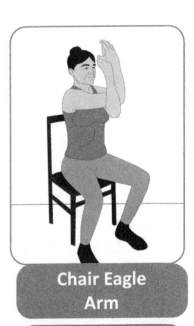

Chair Eagle Arm

Pag 18

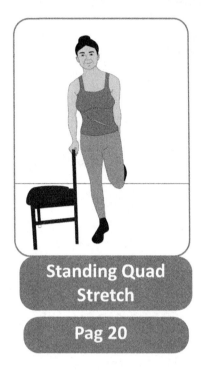

Standing Quad Stretch

Pag 20

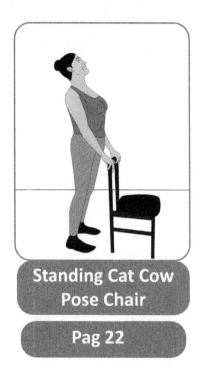

Standing Cat Cow Pose Chair

Pag 22

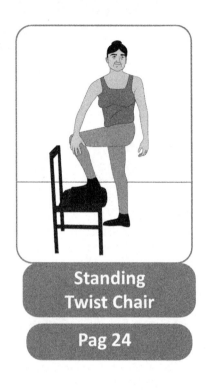

Standing Twist Chair

Pag 24

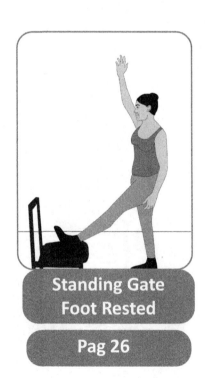

Standing Gate Foot Rested

Pag 26

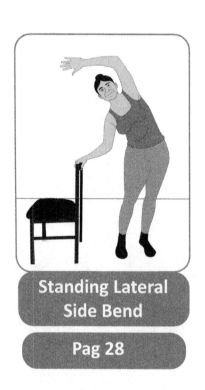

Standing Lateral Side Bend

Pag 28

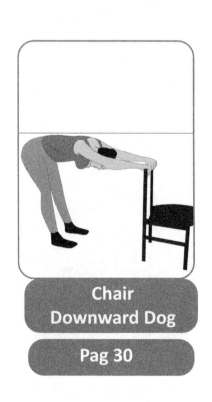

Chair Downward Dog

Pag 30

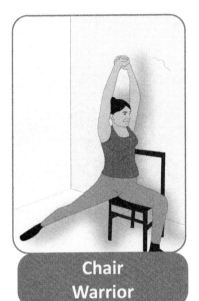

Chair Warrior

Pag 32

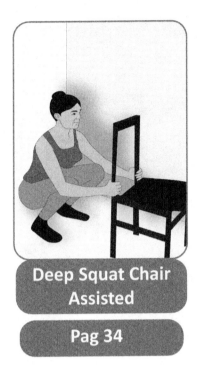

Deep Squat Chair Assisted

Pag 34

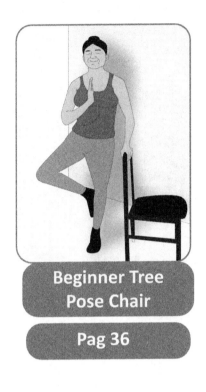

Beginner Tree Pose Chair

Pag 36

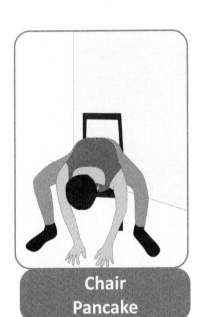

Chair Pancake

Pag 38

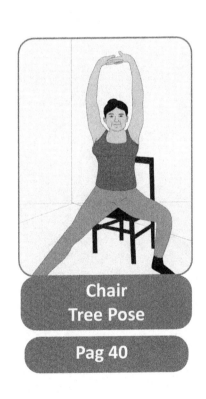

Chair Tree Pose

Pag 40

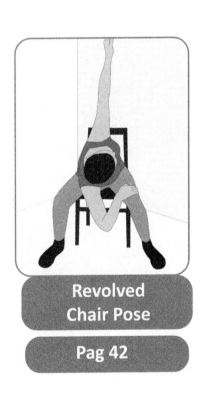

Revolved Chair Pose

Pag 42

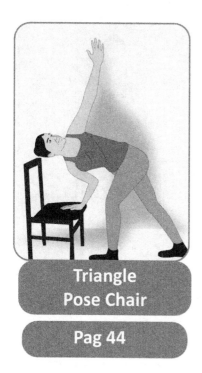

**Triangle
Pose Chair**

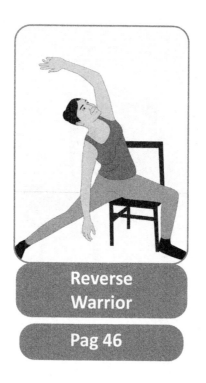

**Reverse
Warrior**

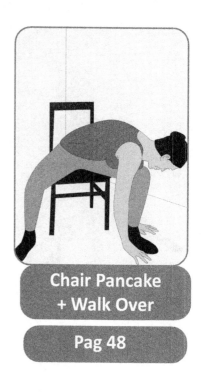

**Chair Pancake
+ Walk Over**

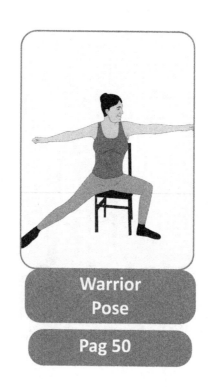

**Warrior
Pose**

FULL BODY TONING

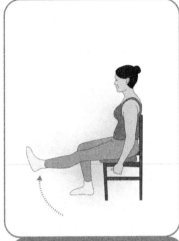

**Seated
Leg Up**

Pag 52

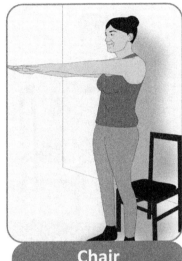

**Chair
Squat**

Pag 54

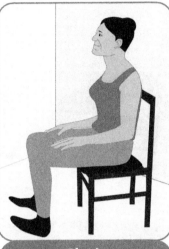

**Chair
Tibialis Raises**

Pag 56

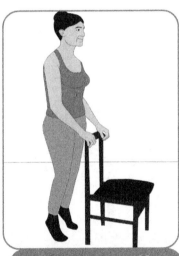

**Standing Calf
Raises Assisted**

Pag 58

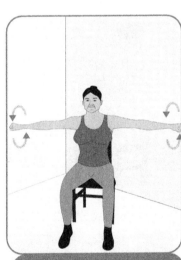

**Chair
Airplane**

Pag 60

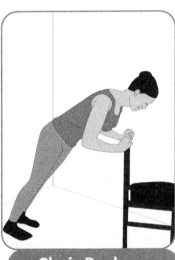

**Chair Push up
Level 1**

Pag 62

X

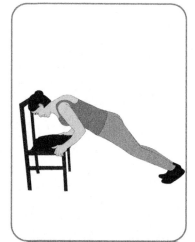

**Chair Push up
Level 2**

Pag 64

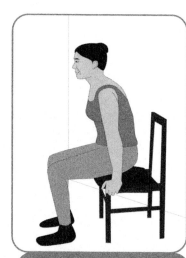

**Chair Assisted
L-Sit Level 1**

Pag 66

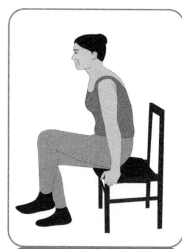

**Chair Assisted
L-Sit Level 2**

Pag 68

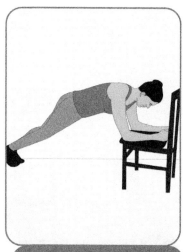

**Chair
Upward Plank**

Pag 70

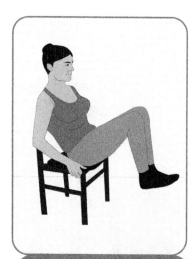

**Seated
Knee-Chest Level 1**

Pag 72

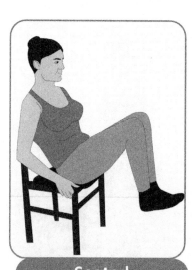

**Seated
Knee-Chest Level 2**

Pag 74

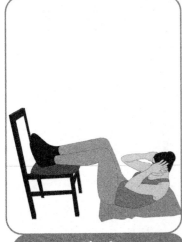

Chair Sit Up

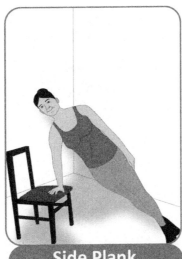

Side Plank Variation Hand Chair

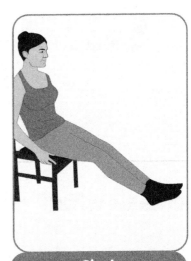

Chair Leg Raises

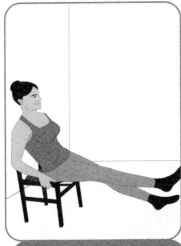

Chair Leg Kick Level 1

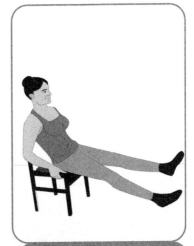

Chair Leg Kick Level 2

Chair Exercises
for Seniors

Guess what? Here's a gift for you

● A special and direct way to text me if you have any questions or just want to say hi!

Don't like texting! No problem! Email me anytime at **avfitness99coaching@gmail.com** ✉️

I'm here to help you with your fitness ! 💪

CHAIR EXERCISES

Chair Exercises for Seniors is a book designed by an experienced personal trainer with exercises and workouts to get stronger, tone your muscles and improve your flexibility at the same time with low-impact exercises.

Additionally, you won't have to worry about anything to get started- all you need is a chair!

Are Chair Exercises Effective?

Short Answer: yes.

Long Answer: exercise does not always mean you have to do extreme activities to strengthen your body, and Chair Exercises prove it.

It is a fantastic practice to help seniors get better physical health through simple ways that are easy to perform and extremely beneficial!

I can assure you that these exercises will make you feel like in your prime years!

BENEFITS FOR SENIORS

Regardless if you are coming back from an injury, you want to tone up your body or simply improve your mobility these exercises have been proven exercises, and this 4-Week method works. Below are the main benefits that you will notice doing Chair Exercises:

• **Pain Relief and Injury Prevention**

This is the first benefit you are going to notice. If you struggle with aching low back, knees, elbows, shoulder or wrist, these exercises will help you tremendously. In fact, they target the muscles around these areas making the joint more secure and stable, decreasing the likelihood of daily-life injuries. This will inevitably make you more confident of your body and increase your self-esteem!

• **Improved Mobility and Balance**

During our lives, we tend to become more sedentary and less active as we age. We will, as a result, become weak and vulnerable because of this weak and fragile body. Chair Exercises are great to strengthen the abs and other muscles to improve your posture and balance.

How are you going to achieve that? In the book, there's a full section related to Core Exercises, particularly designed for seniors with different exercises and levels– and this is something I studied over the last few years for someone like you that might lack experience with exercise or does not have a strong core to begin with.

• **Muscles more Toned and Improved Strength**

Chair Exercises are a wonderful way to improve the tonicity of your muscles all around your body. This is due to its nature and the resistance we place with simply using your bodyweight. Some exercises require strength, balance, and flexibility... Ideal to rediscover the power of your body!

SENIORS' MOTIVATION: THE 5 KEY ASPECTS

1. Develop the habit of exercise.

If you know you are going to work out every day as soon as you wake up, it will become second nature and you will not think about it twice!

Most people made the mistake of not planning their workout during the day. However, in most days you will not feel like exercising, and so you will probably not work out. Planning it in advance helps to stay more consistent,

Here are a few moments in which is great to do the workout:

• After you wake up, whether in the morning or after a nap, if you take them.

• Before you cook meals.

• Before going to sleep (Not recommended for many people as it might keep you up at night, but for some people it is good to release some energy and fall asleep faster).

2. Having a workout notebook.

I am not saying you have to become a fitness fanatic, measuring all your progress meticulously and tracking how you feel after every set.

Simply having a piece of paper that you can use as accountability to see whether you worked out each day can really be helpful.

Simply write down the date and tick a box in case you trained.

Do that for a month and see how many you did. I can guarantee you, based on clients' experiences, that you will feel fulfilled and immensely proud of yourself watching how many days you have been trained, whether you feel like it or not.

3. Think about the results you will obtain.

This is about the effort you put in and the results you get out. Let's assess the differences between the two:

NOT EXERCISING

The cost of not working out are:

- Your health.
- Your overall mood and vitality.
- Your low energy during the day.

The benefits of not exercising are:

- None.

EXERCISING

The cost of exercising is:

- 10-20 min of exercise.

The benefits of exercising are:

- Increased core strength.
- Improved well-being.
- More energy during the day.
- Stronger bones and more toned muscles.
- Increased balance.
- Less risk of injury and joint pain.

Which one would you choose? 10 min of effort or a lifetime of aching and pain? If you are reading this, chances are you made the right choice, and this book will help you in achieving your best self!

4. Give yourself some reward.

Improve in the exercise you struggled last Monday, finishing the workout feeling less tired, being able to walk up the stairs without holding onto any assistance. Take notes of your progress as they will arrive, look back of what you accomplished, and use it as further motivation to exercise even more!

5. Be grateful for it.

There is nothing better than physical exercise and seeing how your body, eventually, adapts to it. Understanding that you are lucky and have the possibility to exercise and move your body is something that will make you feel grateful, and make you feel well and appreciate more what you can do.

You also get the benefits, if you do it long enough, to enjoy the fruit of your hard work...how cool!

HOW TO READ THIS BOOK TO GET THE MOST OUT OF IT

Here, I will show you the best way to read this book. In fact, merely going through pages is not really effective.

I highly recommend you to:

• Start skimming through exercises and get a sense of it. See the differences between them (there are two main sections, one on stretching and poses and the second one on muscle toning for lower body, core and upper body). You might also perform some exercises to get a taste on how they feel whilst doing it.

• Once you get an idea, go to the 4-week plan, and start from there. I would suggest you start from Monday, so let's say you are reading this on Thursday, take the weekend to try out different exercises without any scheme, and start the 4-Week Plan the next Monday!

Note: The 4-Week Plan helped hundreds of seniors as it has been created after training dozens of seniors 1-on-1 and getting feedback from them. The key is the small progression created over time leading to incredible results in just 28 days! However, if you just want to start from performing some exercises without a specific scheme, feel free to do so. Anything but lack of exercise is welcomed!

Extra Tips: The most destructive habit you can have is to think that you have to get fit. Many people approach training with the idea of a certain goal to attain in a specific time. This is great to give you motivation at the beginning. However, when you attain that goal, then what?

At this point, many of my clients stopped training. Waited a few months. And then come back, wishing they had not given up.

The best framework is that you do not train to get fit but simply to stay fit. It is a "Infinite game", and I would highly suggest you to simply wake up every morning and behave as a fit person would do (training, eating right, sleeping well...).

Have as many "fit days" in a row as you can, and you will not even have to worry about the results. They will come 100%!

CHAIR EXERCISES FOR SENIORS STRETCHING POSES

Hand Stretch Pose

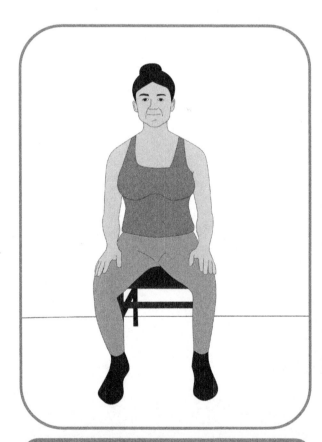

Step 1- Starting position.

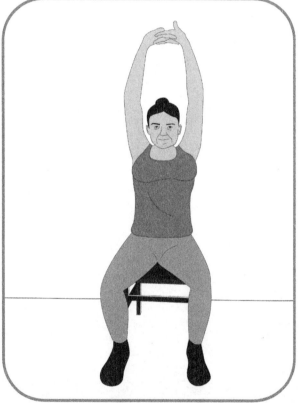

Step 2- Final position with hands over your head.

How to do it:

1. Sit on a chair with back straight, shoulder relaxed and hands on your thighs.

2. Take two deep breaths. Remember to Inhale via your nose in 2-3'', and then exhale through your mouth or nose . Exhale slowly in 4-5''.

3. Initially, inhale and raise your arms in front of you. Keep them straight and lock the fingers to each other. Palms facing in front of you. Exhale softly.

4. Then, as shown in Step 2, inhale and raise your arms over your head. Keep them straight and lock the fingers to each other. Palms facing in front of you. Exhale fully and feel the stretch on your hands and wrist.

Breathing:

Make sure to keep breathing. Breaths will be soft, mostly from your nose. If you feel tight and tense, exhale fully from your mouth.

Note:

Make sure not to lift your shoulders as you do so. This gentle stretch is amazing for your posture as well as wrist and hands' health. You will feel more energized once you do that and with more freedom of movement.

In case you struggle to lift your arms over your head as showed in the illustration, try do lift them as high as you can in a pain-free level. Overtime you will get better.

Neck Side to Side

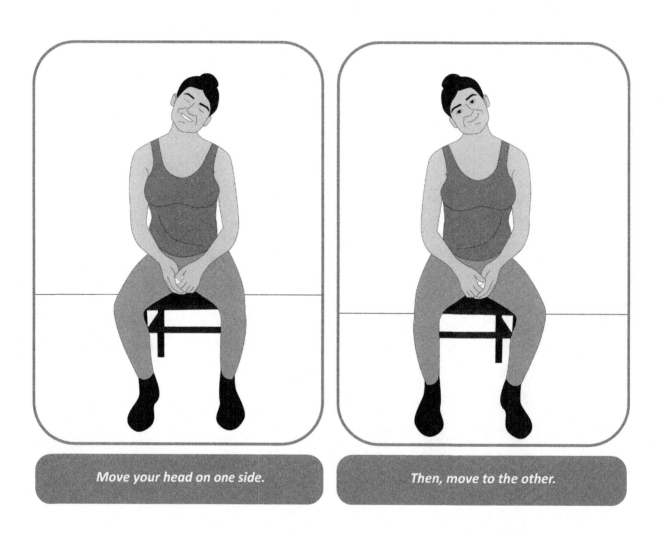

Move your head on one side.

Then, move to the other.

How to do it:

1. Sit comfortably on a chair. Keep your back straight and relax your shoulders. Feet hip width apart flat on the floor and take a deep breath to relax fully.

2. Then, exhale via your nose and move your head to the left side bringing your ear and shoulders close to each other.

3. Then, inhale and come back into the starting position.

4. Repeat on the other side.

Breathing:

Exhale as you move your head to the side and inhale as you come back with your head in resting position.

Note:

Very gentle stretch. As you move your head side to side and feel the stretch on your neck, make sure to keep your shoulders relaxed.

Chair Calf Stretch

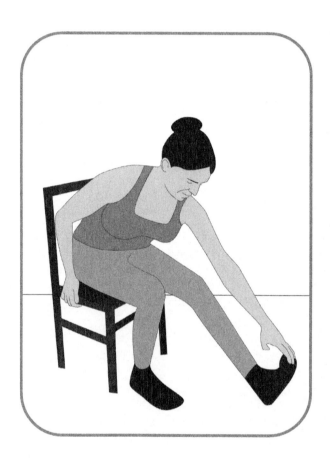

How to do it:

1. Sit comfortably on a chair with feet planted on the floor and upper body relaxed.

2. Extend the left leg so that only the heel is in touch with the floor.

3. Lean forward and extend the left arm towards your foot.

4. By doing this, you will feel a stretch on the back of your lower leg.

5. Hold it for 15'' and then release. Come back into the starting position and repeat on the right side.

Breathing:

During the stretch make sure to keep breathing in a slow and controlled manner. Do not hold your breath as it would tense your body.

Note:

There is no need to try touching your toes with your hand. Go until you feel a stretch and hold that position. Over time your muscle will be able to tolerate more stretch, so that you can go deeper into it. Amazing stretch especially if you have tight calves.

Chair Quad Stretch

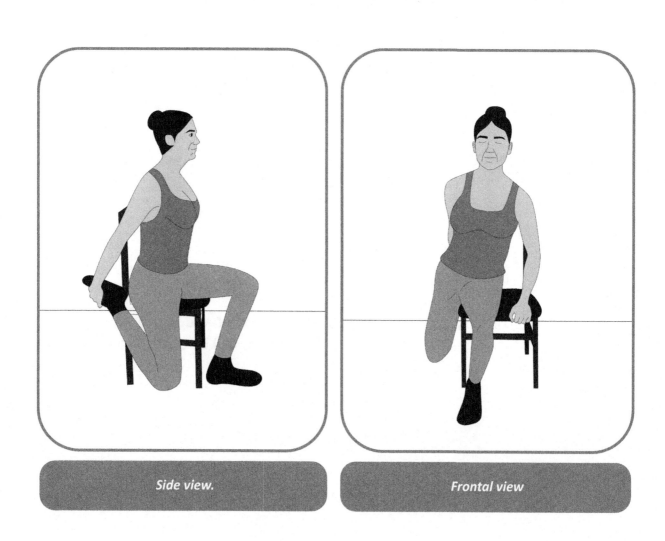

Side view.

Frontal view

How to do it:

1. Sit on a chair keeping your back straight. Only the left glute and back of the thighs are in touch with the chair. The right hip and thighs are hanging out.

2. Make sure that the left knee is a bit away from the chair. Alignment plays a key role in this pose.

3. Grab your right foot with your right hand and point your right knee to the floor if your mobility allows it. Stop the movement once you feel a stretch on your thighs. Hold it for 15'' (Position the left hand on the chair for support if needed).

4. To release, slowly let go of the stretch, come back into the starting position, and repeat on the other side.

Breathing:

During the stretch make sure to keep breathing in a slow and controlled manner. Do not hold your breath as it would tense your body.

Note:

Particularly good to avoid quad stiffness as well as if you experience knee pain. Remember to not push yourself too hard too soon. As soon as you bring your foot and feel a mild stretch, stay there. Over time you will be able to get into a more advanced position. Trust the process!

Triceps Seated Stretch

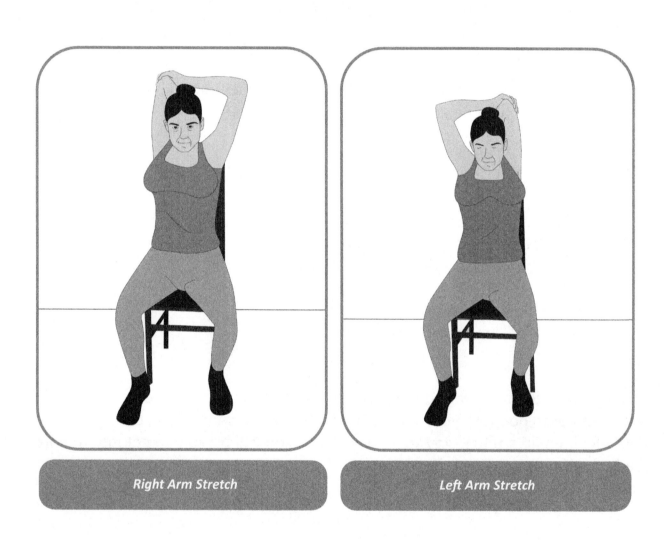

Right Arm Stretch

Left Arm Stretch

How to do it:

1. Sit comfortably with back straight, shoulder relaxed, and feet planted on the floor.

2. Lift your right arm up over your head. Bend it at the elbow so that the right arm is behind your neck.

3. Use the left hand to push the right elbow towards your left side.

4. Hold for 20'' and release. Then, repeat on the other side.

Breathing:

Make sure to breathe slowly and softly, with exhale longer than inhale. Focus on it will improve the stretch's effectiveness.

Note:

Stop and hold the position in which you feel a mild stretch. After a few breaths you will be able to go deeper into the stretch.

One of the best exercises to stretch the back of your arms.

Chair Eagle Arm

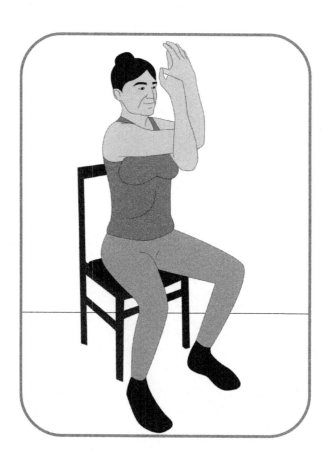

How to do it:

1. Sit comfortably with your back straight and chest up.

2. Take a deep breath while stretching your arms by your sides.

3. After exhaling, bring your arms in front of you, then swing your right arm under your left.

4. The next step is to bend your elbows at 90°, having your forearm up. Then, intertwine your arms. Hold this position for 10-20''.

Breathing:

All the breath in the instructions must be performed slowly. Aim for 2'' for each inhale and 3-4'' for each exhale.

Note:

Amazing stretch for your arms and back of your shoulders.

Standing Quad Stretch

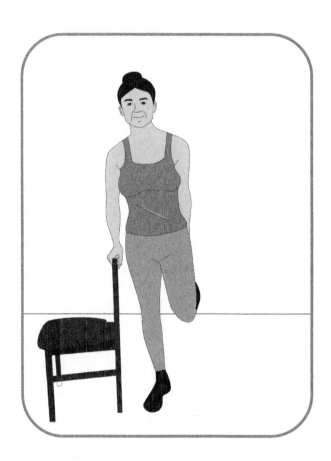

How to do it:

1. Stand alongside the chair's backrest.

2. Place your right hand on the chair for assistance.

3. Lift your left foot and bring it towards your glutes.

4. Grab your left foot with your left hand.

5. Push the foot towards your glutes until you feel a mild stretch on the front of your thighs.

6. Hold it for 10-20'' and repeat on the other side.

Breathing:

Make sure to keep breathing through your nose softly the entire time.

Note:

Highly effective exercise to avoid muscle tightness on the front of your thighs. Also, it works your balance. For an extra challenge try not to hold on to the seat.

Standing Cat Cow Pose Chair

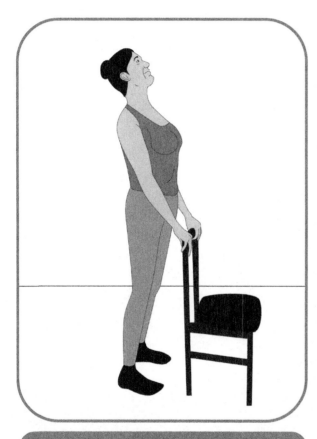

Step 1 - Inhale and open up your chest.

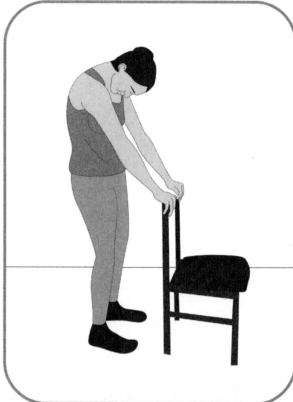

Step 2 - Exhale and bring your chest in.

How to do it:

1. Stand in front of the chair facing the seat.

2. Place your hands on the chair whilst keeping arms and back straight (Try to keep your legs straight too if possible).

3. Inhale and arch your back, opening up your chest for 2-3''.

4. Exhale fully through your mouth and bring your chest in keeping your chin down as you do so. Hold the stretch for 1'' and repeat it 3-6 times.

Breathing:

Inhale via your nose when rounding your back, exhale through your mouth when arching your back.

Note:

Great exercise to mobilize the spine, feel looser in movements, and improve your posture.

Standing Twist Chair

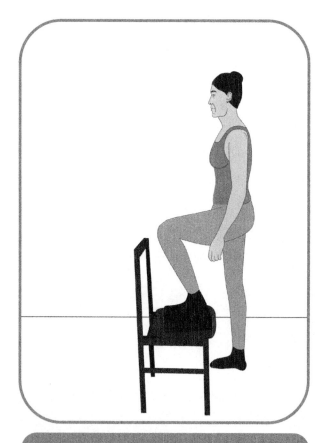

Starting position - Feet on the seat (use a wall for assistance if needed).

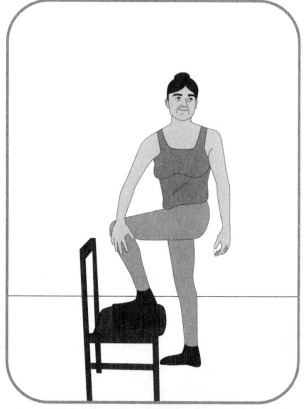

Final position - Twisting your body in the front leg's direction.

How to do it:

1. Stand in front of a chair and place your left leg on top of it. Foot planted on the chair.

2. Rotate your body towards the left leg and bring the right arm on the outside of your left thigh.

3. Hold the position for 5 seconds. Then, release and repeat on the other side.

Breathing:

Make sure to exhale fully once you do this exercise. Inhale via your nose if possible and exhale through your mouth. The exhale is longer than the inhale. Aim for 3 full deep breaths before changing sides.

Note:

This is an amazing twisted stretch for your hips and lower back that can be performed at any level!

Standing Gate Foot Rested

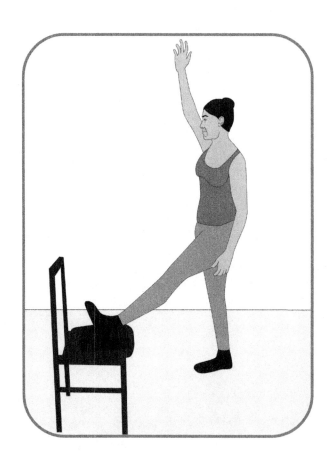

How to do it:

1. Stand alongside a chair, one-arm distance apart.

2. Position your left heel on the chair with leg straight,

3. Inhale and lift your right arm over your head.

4. Exhale deeply and bend down towards the chair, pushing your hips to the right. Your left arm can touch your left leg for assistance.

5. Hold this position for 2-3 deep breaths and repeat on the other side.

Breathing:

No major tips are needed. Make sure to keep breathing once stretching your side abs. This will allow you to get deeper into the stretch.

Note:

Exceptionally good exercise that works on balance and coordination as well as flexibility. Many people experience differences between the sides. If that's you, no worries! It is normal to have one side slightly more coordinated and flexible than the other.

Standing Lateral Side Bend

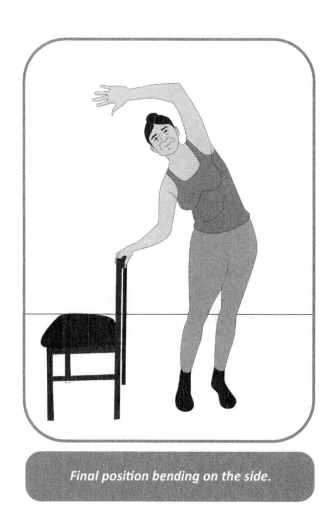

Final position bending on the side.

How to do it:

1. Stand alongside a chair, one-arm distance apart.

2. Place your right hand on the chair's backrest and lift the other arm straight over your head.

3. From there inhale deeply, and then exhale. Once you exhale, bend towards the chair. Get as deep as comfortable into the stretch.

4. Hold the stretch for 2-4 breaths and then exhale and come into standing pose. Repeat on the other side.

Breathing:

Inhale as you lift your arm over your head to start, and then exhale as you bend. Breathe deeply and slowly whilst stretching.

Note:

Focus on your low back and side abdominal muscles whilst holding the position, releasing all the tension in those areas.

Chair Downward Dog

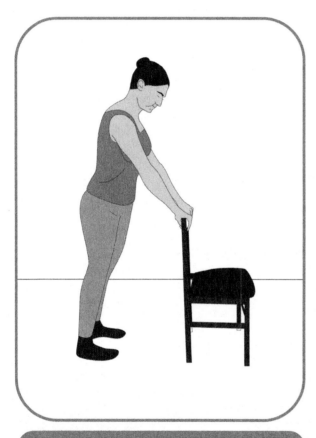

Step 1 - Standing in front of the chair's backrest.

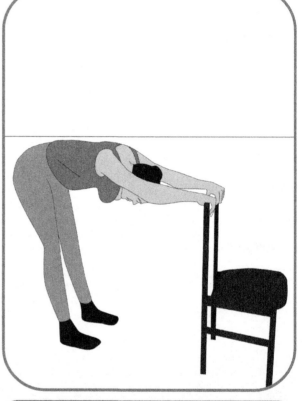

Step 2 - Stretching your shoulder and back leaning forward with back straight.

How to do it:

1. Stand upright and face the seat of your chair one to two feet away from it.

2. Then, bend forward before placing your hands on your chair's seat.

3. To get deeply into the stretch push your glutes back (bending your knee is fine).

4. Take a deep breath holding the pose and then come back into the starting position.

Breathing:

Inhale before bending forward, and then fully exhale once you are stretching your back. Ideally inhale through your nose and exhale through your mouth.

Note:

The further away you go from the chair the deeper you can get into the stretch. Having the trunk parallel to the floor whilst stretching is a very good standard to aim for.

Chair Warrior

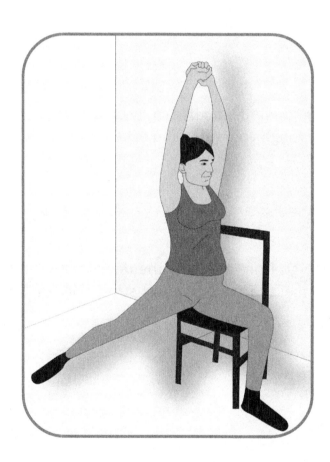

How to do it:

1. Place the left leg in position over the side of the chair while you swing the right leg behind you.

2. Right foot is planted on the floor with the leg straight. Keep your torso facing over the left leg.

3. Then, inhale and lift your arms up towards the ceiling.

4. Hold the stretch for three deep breaths. Then, switch sides.

Breathing:

Make sure to inhale through your nose if possible and exhale through your mouth slowly. This would enhance the efficacy of the exercise.

Note:

Very good exercise for opening up the hips and improving your body awareness. Suitable for beginners too.

Deep Squat Chair Assisted

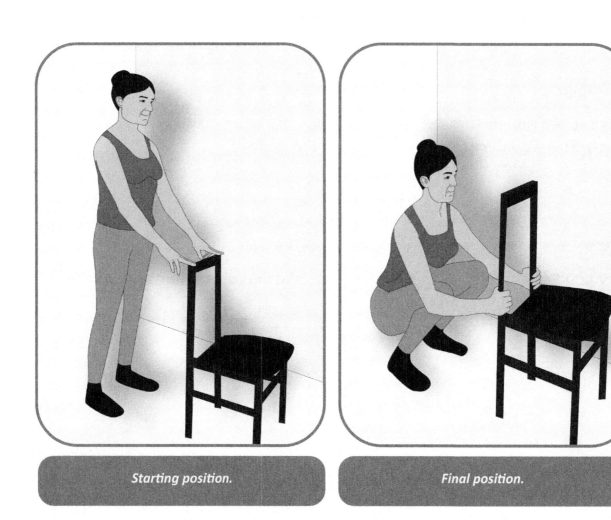

Starting position.

Final position.

How to do it:

1. Position yourself in front of the chair, one-arm distance from it.

2. Inhale and squat down with knees fully bent.

3. Stretch your arms in front of you and hold the chair, for assistance.

4. Take anywhere between 4-6 deep breaths and come back into standing position.

Breathing:

Inhale via your nose and exhale slowly through your mouth.

Note:

If you have major hip and knee pain avoide this exercise for now. You will achieve it in a few weeks if you stick to the other exercises.

When you do it, make sure to fully relax your body whilst exhaling. Go slowly into a squat position to avoid pain or discomfort, if not used to this range of motion. Also, feel free to elevate your heels if it feels more natural. This is a great stretch for your ankles, hip, knees as well as muscle inside of your thighs and glutes...A highly effective exercise.

Beginner Tree Pose Chair

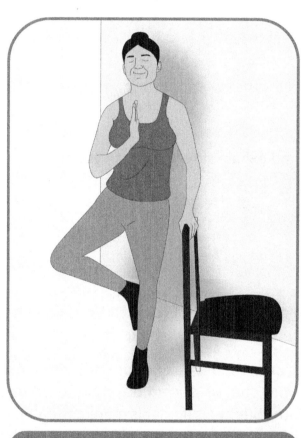

Hold this position for 5" and then repeat on the other side.

How to do it:

1. Stand next to the backrest of the chair with your left hand on it.

2. Slowly shift the weight to the left foot and lift the right foot, moving it against the inside of your left shin.

3. Bring the right palm in front of your chest. If you feel comfortable bring your palms together in front of your chest (in that case, you have to let go of the chair as a support).

4. Hold that position for 5'' and come back into the starting position. Then repeat on the other side.

Breathing:

Make sure to breathe fully, with long inhales and exhales. This would make sure that you are in the present moment, and help you focus on your balance more.

Note:

Focus on spreading your foot on the floor. This will help to balance more easily. Also, this exercise is way more efficient doing it barefoot. For an extra challenge, try closing your eyes and keep the balance!

Chair Pancake

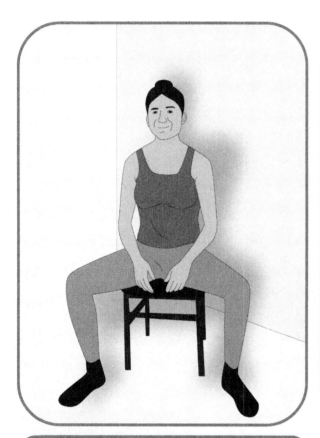

Step 1

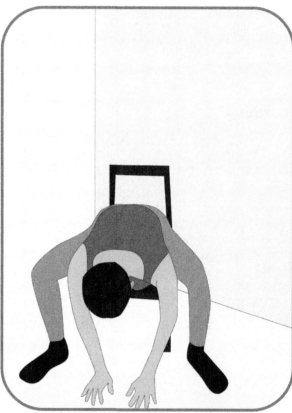

Step 2 - Fold all the way down.

How to do it:

1. Seated in a comfortable position and spread your feet.

2. Fold all the way down whilst keeping your heels on the floor. Ideally hands on the floor.

3. Hold for a second, and then come back into the starting position. Repeat for 3-6 reps.

Breathing:

Inhale before initiating the movement and then exhale once you feel the stretch on your back. Very good to release muscles on your low back and to feel overall less stiff.

Note:

Make sure to go down until comfortable. The images in pictures show what you are going to do in a few weeks from now. If now you cannot get that range of motion, that's fine, do not feel discouraged!

Many of my clients achieved this in less than a month. I am sure you will do it too!

Chair Tree Pose

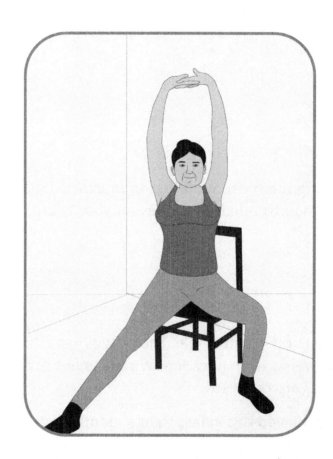

How to do it:

1. Sit at the edge of the chair. Inhale, lift your chest, and exhale drawing your shoulder blades down your back.

2. Extend your right leg straight in front of you and flex your toes pointing at the floor.

3. Open your left leg out to the side, keeping your knee bent and your foot entirely on the floor. Lift your hands to the ceiling with palms intertwined and facing up.

4. Hold that position whilst breathing slowly and controlled. Then release the pose and repeat on the other side.

Breathing:

It is important once you get into the final stretch to exhale and release all the tensions. Most people tend to hold their breath which is counterproductive for the practice.

Note:

No note needed. Start with 3 deep breaths (as mentioned in the plan) and work up to 6 deep breaths, two seconds inhale and four seconds exhaling.

Revolved Chair Pose

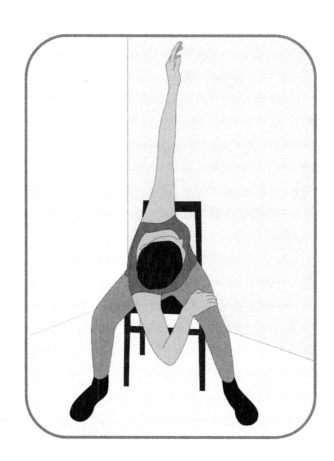

How to do it:

1. Sit down in a comfortable position and spread your legs apart.

2. Then exhale and bend forward as much as comfortable, as you did in Chair Pancake (Two exercises before this one).

3. Then rotate your torso and with your left arm reach up towards the ceiling. Exhale while you do that.

4. Stay in the position for 2-4 breaths. Then slowly come back into the starting position.

5. Repeat on the other side.

Breathing:

Exhaling fully whilst leaning forward and then slowly exhaling is important to optimize the stretch and increase flexibility.

Note:

Even though at first it might be slightly complicated, stick with this exercise. Also make sure not to hold your breath whilst performing it.

Triangle Pose Chair

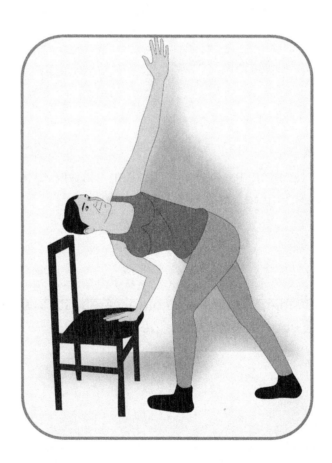

How to do it:

1. Stand in front of a chair with your left leg closer to it.

2. Lean forward keeping your back straight and put your hand on the chair.

3. Rotate your trunk and with your left arm point the ceiling.

4. Hold that position for 2 to 4 deep breaths, release and repeat on the other side.

Breathing:

Make sure to exhale (via nose or mouth) fully once you feel tightness. Common reaction is to hold your breath. This would limit your flexibility and effectiveness of this exercise.

Note:

If you notice any discomfort or a stretch too intense on your abdominal area while doing this stretch, avoid this exercise and try it again in a few weeks, once you will be more used to these exercises.

Reverse Warrior

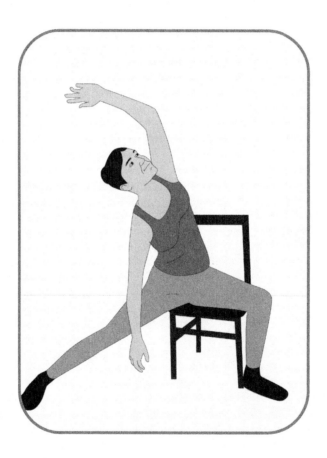

How to do it:

1. Place the left leg in position over the side of the chair while you swing the right leg behind you.

2. Right foot is planted on the floor with right leg straight. Keep your torso facing over the left leg.

3. Inhale and let the right arm come down and lift the left arm over your head. Exhale slowly.

4. Hold the stretch for 5 deep breaths. Then, switch sides.

Breathing:

As you move into this position make sure to never hold your breath as it would tense your body, making it more difficult to execute it correctly.

Note:

This is a great hip opener as well as energy boosters. Make sure both sides get equal stretch while breathing slowly and deeply.

Chair Pancake + Walk Over

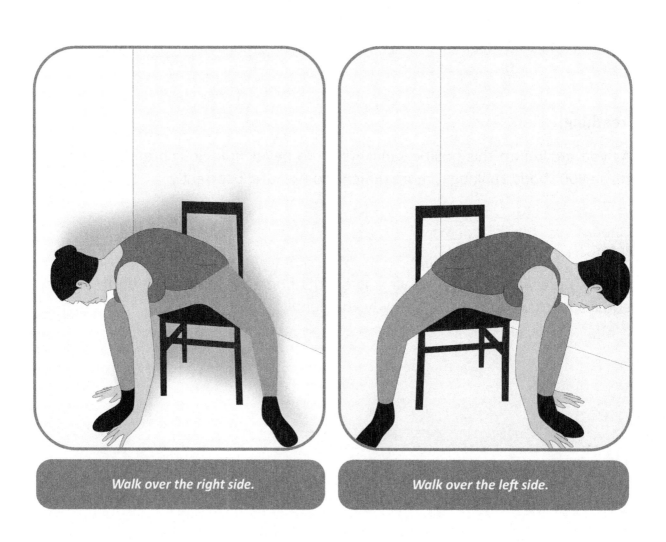

Walk over the right side.

Walk over the left side.

How to do it:

1. Seated in a comfortable position and spread your feet.

2. Fold all the way down whilst keeping your heels on the floor. Ideally hands on the floor.

3. Hold for a second, and then move your arms towards one leg. Then move to the other.

4. Lastly, come back into the starting position. Repeat for the desired reps.

Breathing:

Inhale before initiating the movement and then exhale once you feel the stretch on your back.

Note:

Make sure to go down until comfortable. The images in pictures show what you are going to do in a few weeks from now. If now you cannot get that range of motion, that's fine, do not feel discouraged! Many of my clients achieved this in less than 2 months. I am sure you will do it too!

Warrior Pose

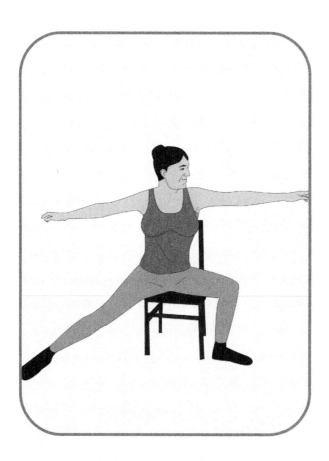

How to do it:

1. Sit on the edge of the chair with your back straight, relax your shoulders. Take a deep breath.

2. Open your left leg so that it is parallel to the backrest.

3. Then, extend the right leg diagonally with foot planted on the floor, as shown in the image.

4. Now lift the left arm on the side pointing forward, and with your gaze look at your fingers.

5. Do the opposite movement with the right arm.

6. Hold this position for 2-3 breaths, release and repeat on the other side.

Breathing:

Make sure to exhale via your mouth if possible. Exhale is always longer than inhale.

Note:

Once you lift your arms be aware of keeping your shoulders relaxed and back straight.

FULL BODY TONING

Seated Leg Up

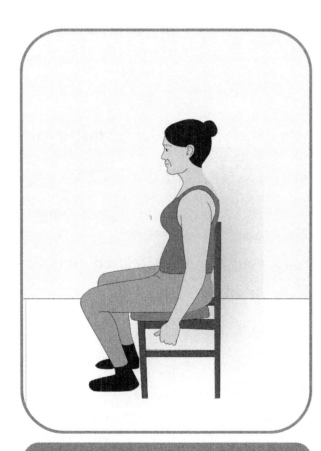

Step 1 - Sit comfortably on a chair.

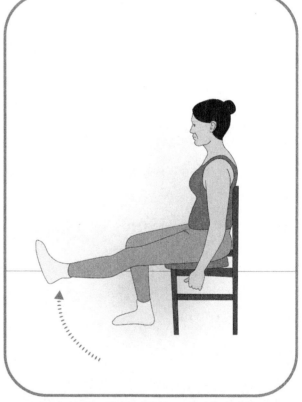

Step 2 - Lift one leg with shin parallel to the floor.

How to do it:

1. Sit on a chair in a comfortable position.

2. Start with one leg and lift it all the way up, with shin parallel to the floor.

3. Hold it for 1'' and then come back down. Repeat for the desired reps and then do it with the other leg.

Breathing:

Exhale through your mouth as you lift the leg straight in front of you and inhale via your nose as you lower down into the initial position.

Note:

This is a great exercise to strengthen the muscle on your thighs, and also to work on your knees. In fact, doing this movement pain-free is a great indicator of your knee health.

Chair Squat

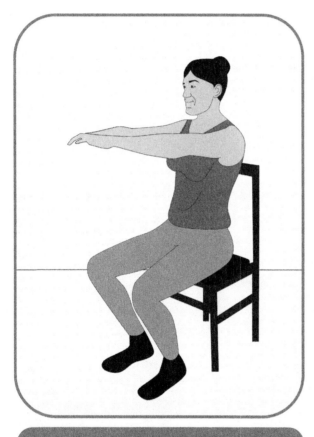

Starting position

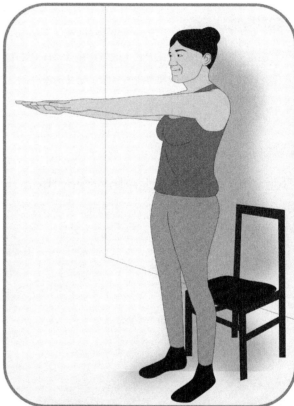

Final Position

How to do it:

1. Sit comfortably on a chair with back straight and arms straight in front of you.

2. Stand up by pushing your feet on the floor. Keep your arms in the same starting position.

3. Hold half a second the standing position and come back into the starting position. Repeat for the desired reps.

Breathing:

Exhale via your nose or mouth as you stand up and inhale as you come back into starting position (seated).

Note:

Joint-friendly exercise that will be amazing to build toned thighs and also help you perform daily movements with ease.

Chair Tibialis Raises

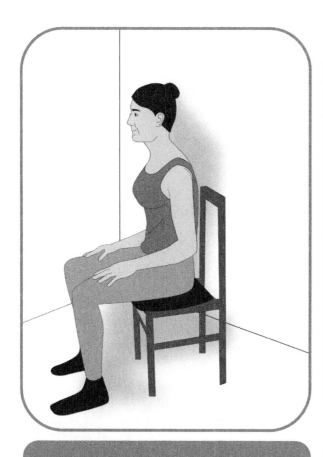

Step 1

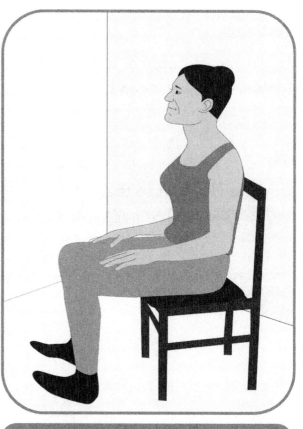

Step 2 – lift your toes as high as you can.

How to do it:

1. Sit comfortably in a chair with your back straight without resting it on the back rest.

2. Knee bent at 90° and the sole of the foot rested on the floor.

3. Lift your toes as high as you can and hold that contraction for 1''.

4. Come back into the starting position and repeat for the desired reps.

Breathing:

Not really necessary in this exercise to focus on breathing based on the execution. Make sure to breathe slowly and controlled without holding your breath, common for some people when exercising.

Note:

Great exercise that is going to work the front muscle of your shins. Also, it is great to avoid ankle injury.

Standing Calf
Raises Assisted

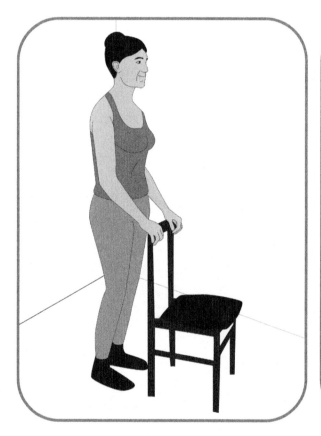
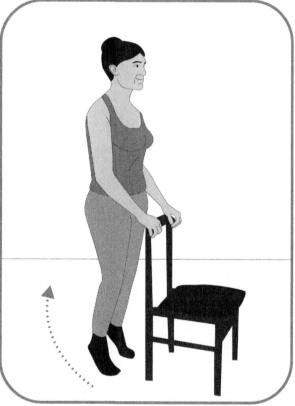

How to do it:

1. Stand behind the chair and put your hands on the chair's backrest for assistance.

2. Lift your heels as high as you can and hold that calf contraction for 1''.

3. Come back into the starting position and repeat for the desired sets.

Breathing:

Not really necessary in this exercise to focus on breathing based on the execution. Make sure to breathe slowly and controlled without holding your breath, common for some people when exercising.

Note:

You have to lift your entire bodyweight with your feet (even though you have assistance for balance). Great exercise to avoid ankle injuries and for stronger feet.

Chair Airplane

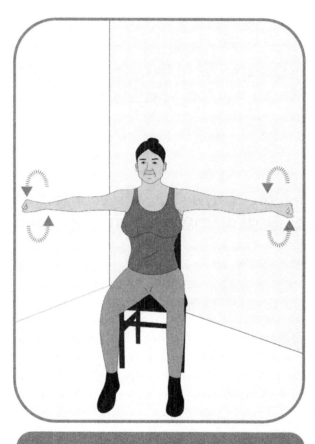

Make small circles with your arms.

How to do it:

1. Sit on a chair and relaxed your upper body exhaling fully.

2. Lift your arms on the side and keep your fists closes.

3. Then, perform small circles with your arms straight.

Breathing:

Make sure not to hold your breath and keep breathing softly whilst doing circles with your arms.

Note:

Keep your shoulders relaxed and far from your ears. This is an amazing exercise to tone up your arms and shoulders.

Chair Push up Level 1

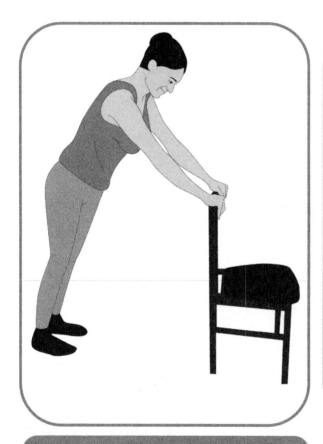

(Really recommended to find a
stable set up or use a table)

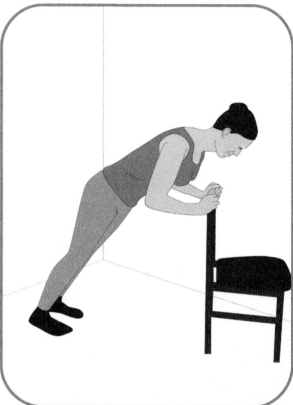

Lower down using your arms and
keeping your body straight. then push
back into starting position.

How to do it:

1. Stand in front of the backrest of the chair, two feet away from it.

2. Lean forward and put your hands shoulder-width apart on the back rest. (Go on the ball of your feet if that's comfortable for you, otherwise stay with feet planted on the floor.)

3. Go down slowly until your elbows are bent at 90° whilst keeping your body straight.

4. Then push back up and come back into the starting position. As you do so you will feel the back of your arm and your chest working.

5. Repeat for the desired sets.

Breathing:

Inhale via your nose as you come down, and exhale with your nose or mouth as you push back up.

Note:

If you want to do this exercise, place the seat against the wall or a solid platform so that it is not going to move as you perform the movement. It is the second most advanced exercise and you do not have necessarily do it. From the client I have in person, only less than 5% of over 60 can do this.

Attempt it only if the set-up is safe!

Chair Push up Level 2

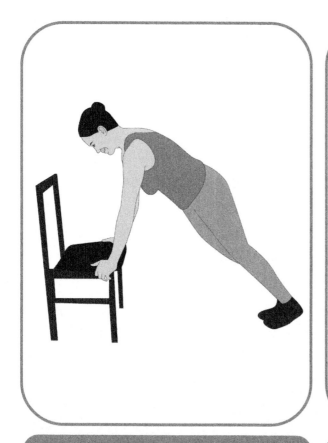

(Make sure chair is firm and not moving)

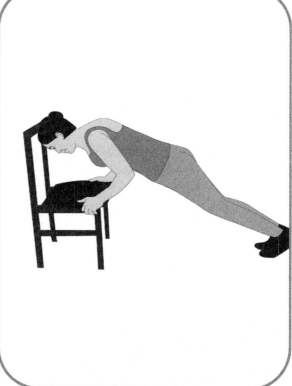

Perform a pushup, going down as long as you feel comfortable without any risk or discomfort.

How to do it:

1. Stand in front of the chair, three to five feet away from it.

2. Lean forward and put your hands shoulder-width apart on the seat. (Go on the ball of your feet if that's comfortable for you, otherwise stay with feet planted on the floor.)

3. Go down slowly until your elbows are bent at 90° whilst keeping your body straight.

4. Then push back up and come back into the starting position. As you do so you will feel the back of your arm and your chest working.

5. Repeat for the desired sets

Breathing:

Inhale via your nose as you come down, and exhale with your nose or mouth as you push back up.

Note:

Very advanced exercise, so approach it with caution.

Make sure to keep your body straight whilst doing the movement. This is an amazing exercise to work your core as well as your arms, shoulders, and chest.

As for the previous exercise, firstly make sure the set-up is safe. This is the most advanced exercise in the book, so you do not really have to do it. Just two seniors I train in person out of many dozens can do this.

Please attempt only in a safe environment and if you feel ready, otherwise wait a few more weeks before trying it!

Chair Assisted L-Sit Level 1

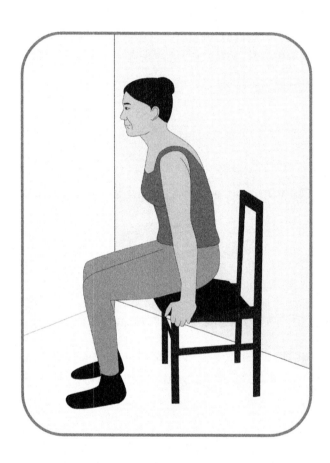

How to do it:

1. Sit with your back straight at the edge of the chair with hands at the sides of the chair for stability.

2. Lift your glutes from the seat by pushing with your hands on the seat.

3. Hold that position with arms straight and hips lifted up for the desired number of seconds (60'' would be amazing).

Breathing:

Make sure not to hold your breath as it will make it more difficult. Breath softly and slowly.

Note:

Make sure to push your shoulders down. This exercise not only is going to work your arms but also it is going to tone up the muscles on your stomach.

Chair Assisted L-Sit Level 2

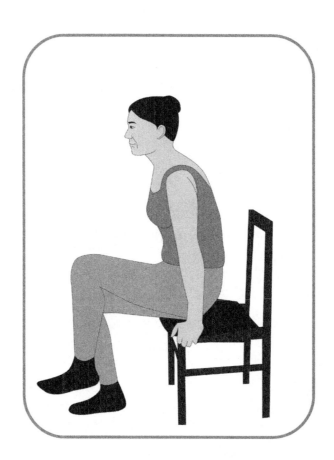

How to do it:

1. Sit with your back straight at the edge of the chair with hands at the sides of the chair for stability.

2. Lift your glutes from the seat by pushing with your hands on the seat.

3. Also, lift one foot off the floor, whilst keeping your knees bent.

4. Hold that position with arms straight and hips lifted up for the desired number of seconds (60'' would be amazing). Then, repeat switching legs.

Breathing:

Make sure not to hold your breath as it will make it more difficult. Breath softly and slowly.

Note:

Unlike Chair Assisted L-Sit Level 1 this is going to put even more tension on your arms as you would only have one foot supporting you!

This is quite advanced, so make sure to master the previous exercise before doing this. It can be quite challenging especially if you carry lot of weight.

Chair Upward Plank

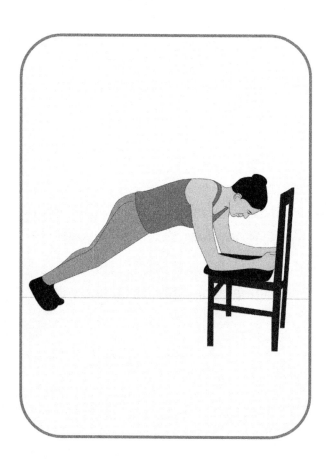

How to do it:

1. Stand in front of a chair.

2. Bend forward to place your forearm on the chair.

3. Then, move your feet backward so you have straight legs.

4. Make sure to lift your glute so your body is a perfect line.

5. Keep that position for a few breaths and then release.

Breathing:

Make sure not to hold your breath whilst holding the position. Keep breathing regularly.

Note:

This is an amazing exercise to work on your core, coordination, and posture. It's not easy at first but definitely an exercise I recommend to you!

As mentioned for the Chair Push-up before doing it make sure the seat is stable and it is not going to move. Remember that safety in the execution is the first parameter, and you do not have to risk your health! I always put the seat against the wall when working with clients. This way the set-up is very stable and safe.

Seated Knee-Chest Level 1

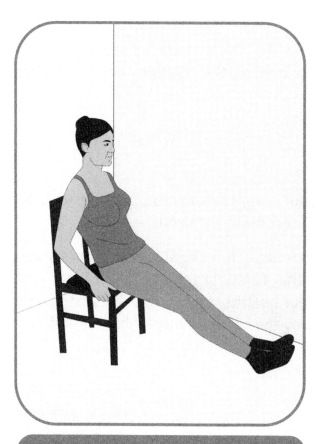

Step 1 - Legs straight in front of you with heels on the floor.

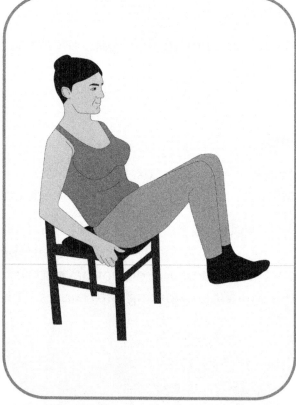

Step 2 - Tuck your knees towards your chest (be gentle, do not overdo it).

How to do it:

1. Sit with your back straight at the edge of the chair with hands at the sides of the chair for stability.

2. Put both feet out in front of the body, point the toes upwards and maintain the heels on the ground.

3. Lift both legs closer to the body while bending the knee. Aim to lift your knee as close as possible to your chest.

4. Perform the movement in the opposite motion (straightening legs) letting your feet touch the floor.

5. Repeat for the mentioned reps.

Breathing:

As you bring your knee towards the chest exhale. Inhale when straightening your leg.

Note:

Make sure to hold tight the chair with your hands. When doing step 3 it is normal to lean backward with your body. Great exercise for your core and overall coordination. Once you master this do the variation in the following page. You do not have necessary to start bringing your knees all the way up as showed. Start with just a little bit of range of motion, and build from there, as showed later in the 4-week plan! No rush of the progress, plenty of people started without even being able to do this and in a matter of a few weeks they were doing it for reps!

Seated Knee-Chest Level 2

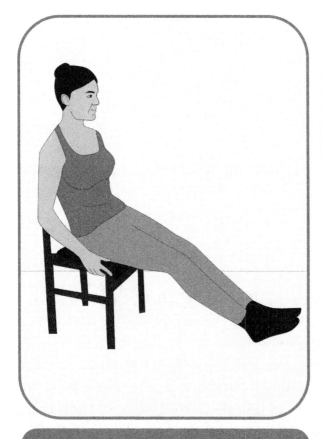

Step 1 - Start with legs straight and heels NOT touching the floor. Legs suspended.

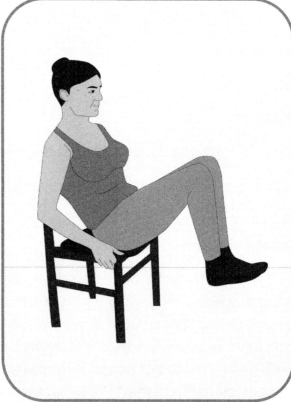

Step 2 - Tuck your knees towards your chest (be gentle, do not overdo it)

How to do it:

1. Sit with your back straight at the edge of the chair .with hands on the sides of the chair for stability.

2. Put both feet out in front of the body and point the toes upwards.

3. Lift both legs closer to the body while bending the knees. Aim to lift your knees as close as possible to your chest.

4. Perform the movement in the opposite motion (straightening legs without letting your feet touch the floor).

5. Repeat for the desired reps.

Breathing:

As you bring your knees towards the chest exhale. Inhale when straightening your legs.

Note:

When doing step 3 it will be natural to lean slightly back with your body. Do Level 1 (previous exercise) if this variation is too difficult. Master the previous one and come back here in a few weeks!

Chair Sit Up

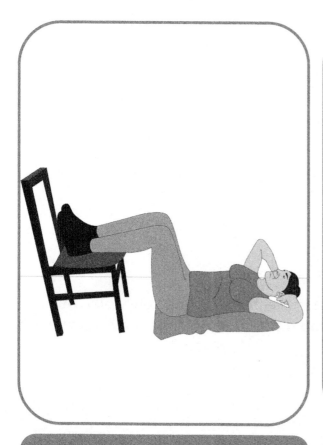

Starting position

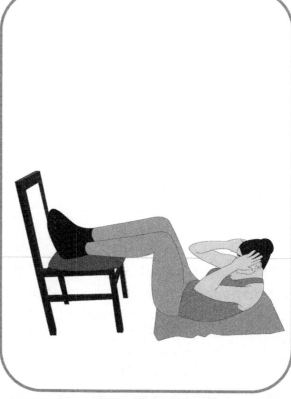

Final position – keep lower back on the floor and lift only upper back to contract your abs.

How to do it:

1. Lay down on the floor with your lower leg resting on the chair and knees bent at 90°.

2. Bring your hands together behind the head, in contact with the floor.

3. Lift your head, neck, and upper back, curling towards the chair. Exhale as you do so.

4. Hold the contraction for half a second and come back into starting position.

5. Repeat for the desired reps.

Breathing:

As you lift your upper back exhale from your mouth, inhale as you come back into a lying position.

Note:

Make sure to always keep your lower back on the floor. By doing that, you will avoid any low back pain or soreness and only focus on working your abdominal muscles. However, if you feel any discomfort laying down feel free to skip this exercise and try it again later on.

Side Plank Variation
Hand Chair

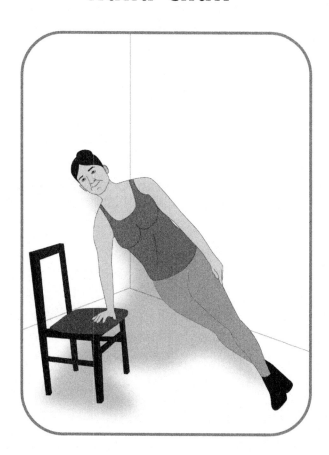

How to do it:

1. Stand alongside the seat of a chair and put your right hand on it with your arm straight.

2. Put your outside of your right foot on the floor, with the left foot next to it for assistance.

3. Try to keep your body as a straight line (do not lift the hip too much or too little).

4. Keep the left arm on your side.

5. Hold that position for the mentioned hold. Goal is to do it for 60'' (that would be very good!) and repeat on the other side.

Breathing:

Make sure to keep inhaling and exhaling slowly and deeply once holding the position.

Note:

Very advanced exercise! It might take a bit longer than expected before doing it ease will good technique as showed.

Keep your chest opened whilst in position and make sure you feel it on your arms and side abs. This is an amazing exercise to have a strong core and good balance that will help you in any activity during the day.

Remember to make sure the seat is stable. I always recommend having it against a wall or a solid platform, so it is not going to move.

Chair Leg Raises

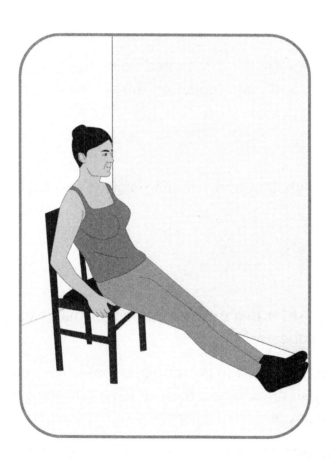

How to do it:

1. Sit on a chair comfortably with your back straight and chest up.

2. Hold with your hands the sit and straighten the legs in front of you.

3. Now lift your foot a few inches from the floor. You are now going to feel a contraction on your thighs and lower abs.

4. Hold for the desired seconds (mentioned in the workout routines) and then release.

Breathing:

Keep breathing. Once you will hold the contraction it will be natural for some people to hold their breath. Keep inhaling via your nose and exhaling through your mouth (or nose) to improve your performance.

Note:

Great core exercises. To make it easier lean backward with your body. For the future, to make it more difficult, simply lift your legs a bit more whilst keeping them straight.

Chair Leg Kick Level 1

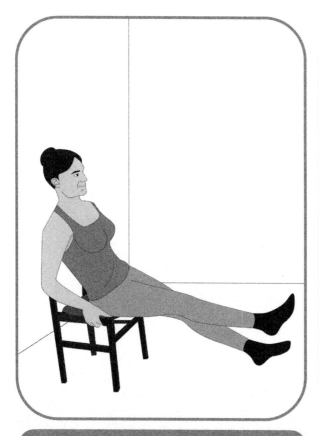

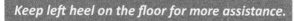
Keep left heel on the floor for more assistance.

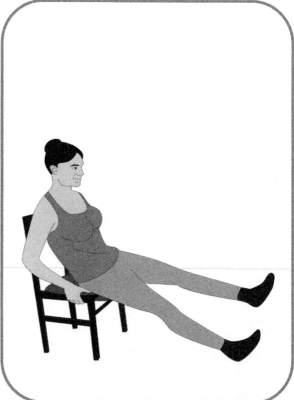
Keep right heel on the floor for more assistance.

How to do it:

1. Sit with your back straight at the edge of the chair with hands at the sides of the chair for stability.

2. Put both feet out in front of the body and point the toes upwards. Lean slightly backward to stabilize yourself.

3. Lift one leg up as high as you can (ideally at hips level) without moving your upper body. The heel of the non-working leg touches the floor for assistance.

4. Slowly lower the leg back to starting position then switch with the other leg.

Breathing:

Make sure not to hold your breath as it will make it more difficult.

Note:

Do Leg Kick Level 2 (following page) if this is too easy.

Chair Leg Kick Level 2

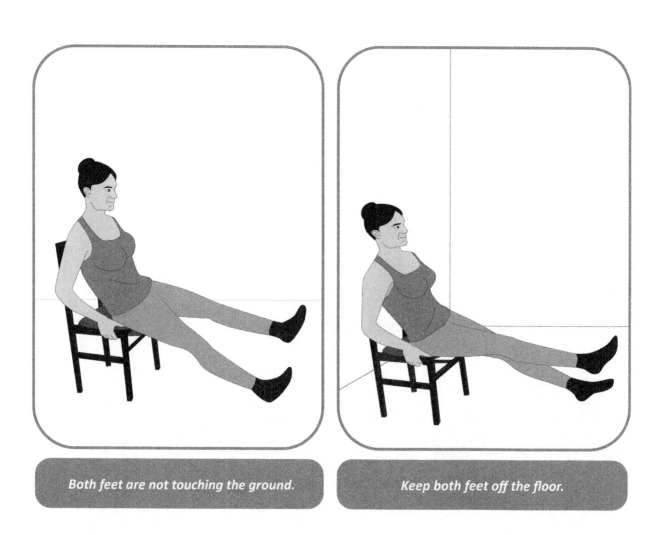

Both feet are not touching the ground.

Keep both feet off the floor.

How to do it:

1. Sit with your back straight at the edge of the chair with hands at the sides of the chair for stability.

2. Put both feet out in front of the body and point the toes upwards. Lean slightly backward to stabilize yourself.

3. Lift one leg up as high as you can (ideally at hips level) without moving your upper body. The other leg is not touching the floor, but it is slightly elevated.

4. Slowly lower the leg back to starting position then switch with the other leg.

Breathing:

Make sure not to hold your breath as it will make it more difficult.

Note:

Do Leg Kick Level 1 (previous exercise) before doing this. Step by step you will get to this exercise, and you will feel (and be) extraordinarily strong!

4-WEEK WORKOUT ROUTINE

This is a 28-Day workout routine. Each day of the week you will be performing different exercises.

By the end of it:

• You will feel energized.

Full Body routines will not only increase your strength and flexibility but also your body will adapt to perform better to tackle daily life activities.

• You will be stronger.

By applying the sets and reps given week after week you will be surprised by how much you can do in such a brief period of time!

• You will feel your body 20 years younger.

Not only strength and mobility, but also cardiovascular exercises! At the end of each workout, there will be a more intense exercise to bring your heart rate up, making your heart stronger too, and feeling fantastic after each session!

Try it yourself!

Notes

• When 2 or more sets for exercise are mentioned, rest anywhere between 10'' and 60'' before starting the new set. Some exercises you will find easy and do not need much rest in between sets, while others it will require a little break.

• This challenge helped 50+ seniors getting fitter, stronger and

with less pain in less than 4 weeks. However, you might not progress as quickly as the progressions showed. Feel free to repeat some sessions. For example, you might want to stick with Week 1 for two to three weeks. Then, when you feel comfortable you jump to Week 2.

• Also, keep in mind that this 28-day challenge is a particularly good challenge for most seniors. I have proven these exact progressions with dozens of people over 60 and it worked well every time! However, if you think this is too challenging or not challenging enough, feel free to adjust the sets and reps based on your current fitness levels!

• I am sure you will be able to do all the exercises. However, make sure to read the notes of each one of them to avoid injury or discomfort. The only two exercises that are very advanced and only a few seniors were able to do it (based on my experience in training many in 1-on-1 sessions) are Side Plank and Push up, both using a chair.

Those two are great exercises that will help you have a better posture and an amazing upper body strength. However, make sure to have a safe set up first (in fact, if you try doing pushups just putting your hands on the chair's backrest and lowering down is a very unsafe exercise!)

I recommend you setting up a chair against the wall in those two exercises making sure that the chair is firm, and it does not move.

However, feel free to skip those two exercises if you feel unsure...You can get remarkable results with all the other ones!

WEEK 01

MONDAY

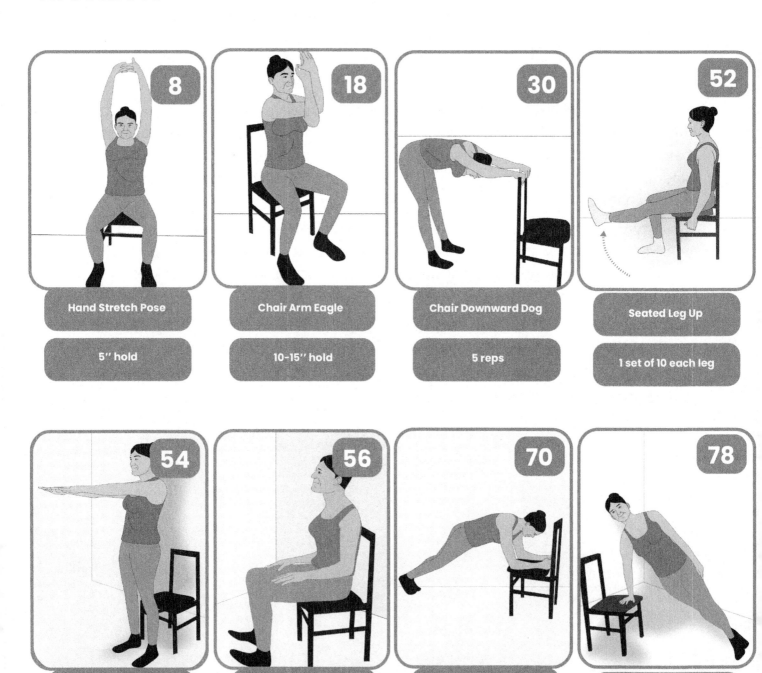

8
Hand Stretch Pose
5'' hold

18
Chair Arm Eagle
10-15'' hold

30
Chair Downward Dog
5 reps

52
Seated Leg Up
1 set of 10 each leg

54
Chair Squat
2 sets of 10

56
Chair Tibialis Raises
2 sets of 10

70
Chair Upward Plank
3 sets of 10''

78
Side Plank Variation
Hand Chair (OPTIONAL)
1 set of 10'' each side

TUESDAY

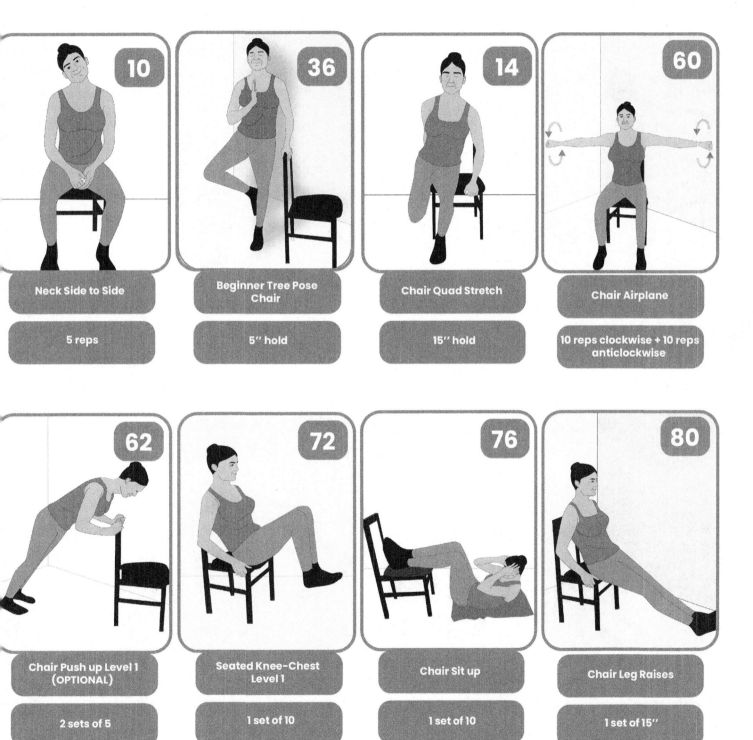

Neck Side to Side	**10**
5 reps	

Beginner Tree Pose Chair	**36**
5" hold	

Chair Quad Stretch	**14**
15" hold	

Chair Airplane	**60**
10 reps clockwise + 10 reps anticlockwise	

Chair Push up Level 1 (OPTIONAL)	**62**
2 sets of 5	

Seated Knee-Chest Level 1	**72**
1 set of 10	

Chair Sit up	**76**
1 set of 10	

Chair Leg Raises	**80**
1 set of 15"	

WEEK 01

WEDNESDAY

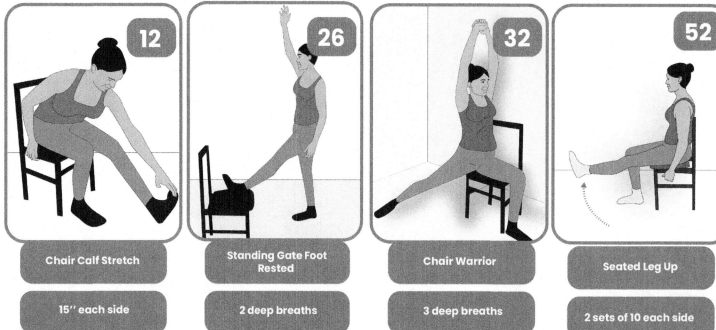

12	**26**	**32**	**52**
Chair Calf Stretch	**Standing Gate Foot Rested**	**Chair Warrior**	**Seated Leg Up**
15" each side	2 deep breaths	3 deep breaths	2 sets of 10 each side

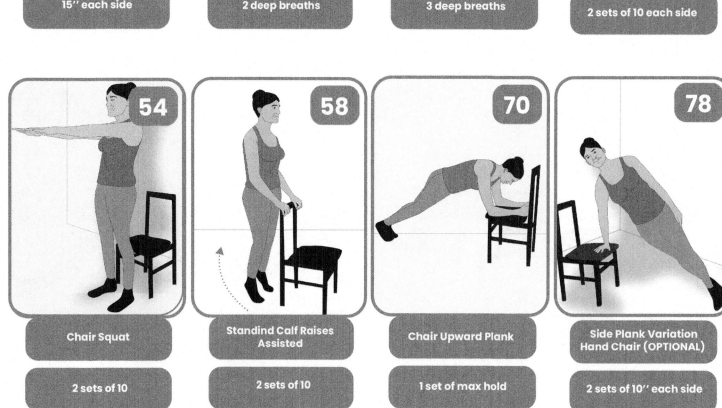

54	**58**	**70**	**78**
Chair Squat	**Standind Calf Raises Assisted**	**Chair Upward Plank**	**Side Plank Variation Hand Chair (OPTIONAL)**
2 sets of 10	2 sets of 10	1 set of max hold	2 sets of 10" each side

WEEK 01

THURSDAY

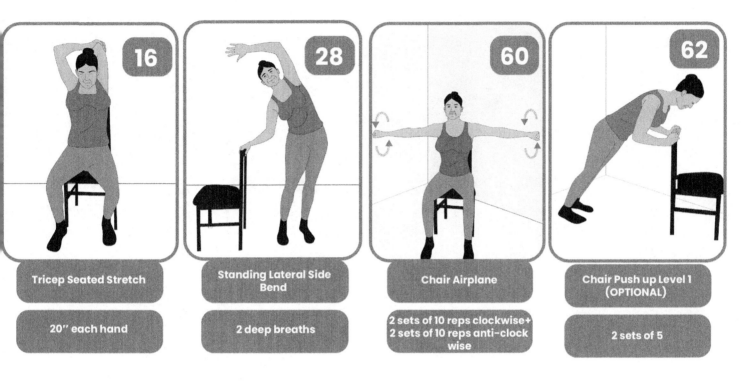

16 — Tricep Seated Stretch — 20" each hand

28 — Standing Lateral Side Bend — 2 deep breaths

60 — Chair Airplane — 2 sets of 10 reps clockwise+ 2 sets of 10 reps anti-clock wise

62 — Chair Push up Level 1 (OPTIONAL) — 2 sets of 5

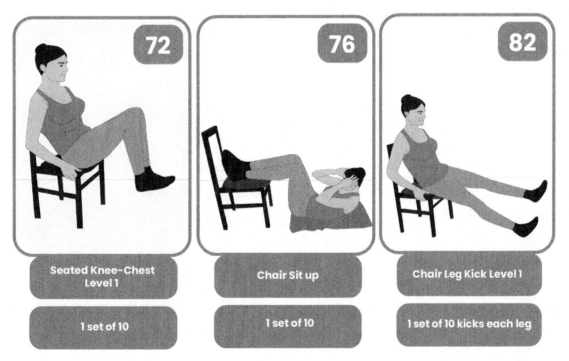

72 — Seated Knee-Chest Level 1 — 1 set of 10

76 — Chair Sit up — 1 set of 10

82 — Chair Leg Kick Level 1 — 1 set of 10 kicks each leg

FRIDAY

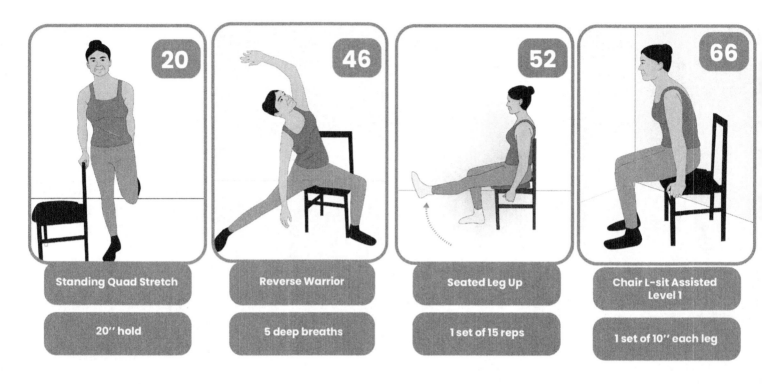

20
Standing Quad Stretch
20″ hold

46
Reverse Warrior
5 deep breaths

52
Seated Leg Up
1 set of 15 reps

66
Chair L-sit Assisted Level 1
1 set of 10″ each leg

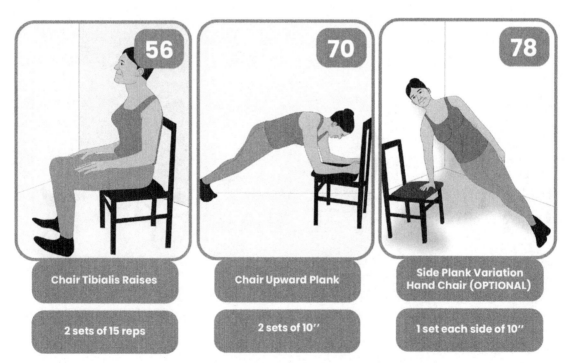

56
Chair Tibialis Raises
2 sets of 15 reps

70
Chair Upward Plank
2 sets of 10″

78
Side Plank Variation Hand Chair (OPTIONAL)
1 set each side of 10″

SATURDAY

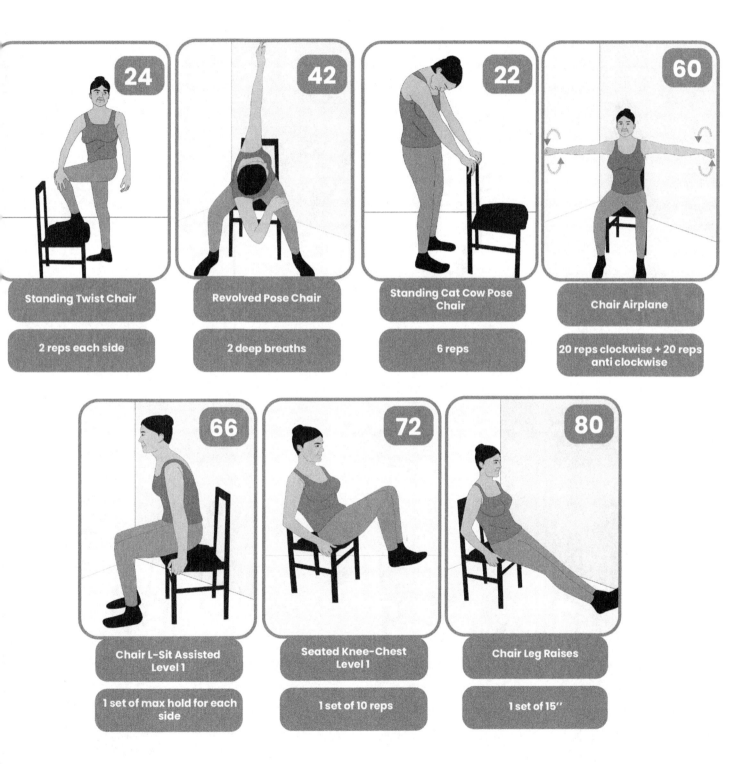

Standing Twist Chair

24

2 reps each side

Revolved Pose Chair

42

2 deep breaths

Standing Cat Cow Pose Chair

22

6 reps

Chair Airplane

60

20 reps clockwise + 20 reps anti clockwise

Chair L-Sit Assisted Level 1

66

1 set of max hold for each side

Seated Knee-Chest Level 1

72

1 set of 10 reps

Chair Leg Raises

80

1 set of 15''

SUNDAY: REST DAY

MONDAY

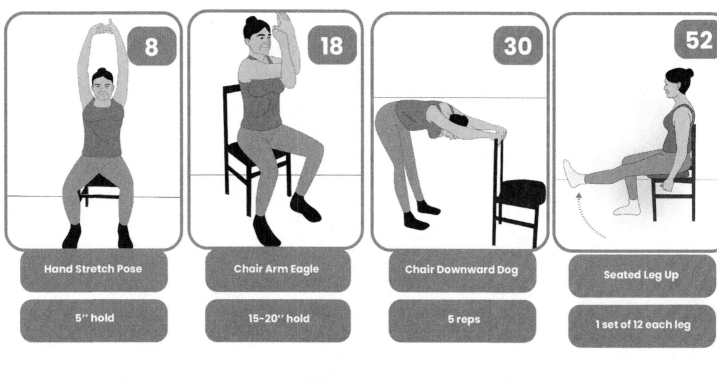

8 Hand Stretch Pose — 5" hold

18 Chair Arm Eagle — 15–20" hold

30 Chair Downward Dog — 5 reps

52 Seated Leg Up — 1 set of 12 each leg

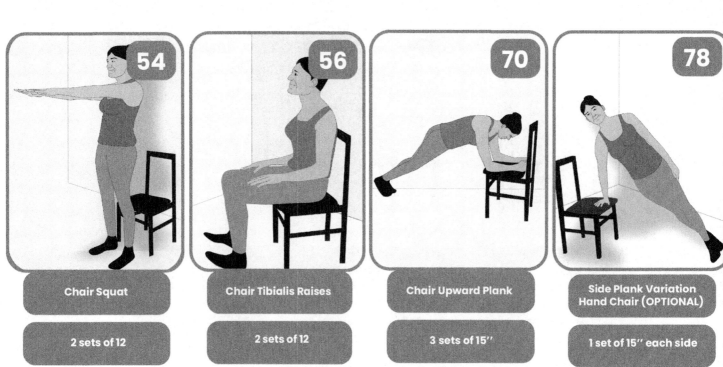

54 Chair Squat — 2 sets of 12

56 Chair Tibialis Raises — 2 sets of 12

70 Chair Upward Plank — 3 sets of 15"

78 Side Plank Variation Hand Chair (OPTIONAL) — 1 set of 15" each side

WEEK 02

TUESDAY

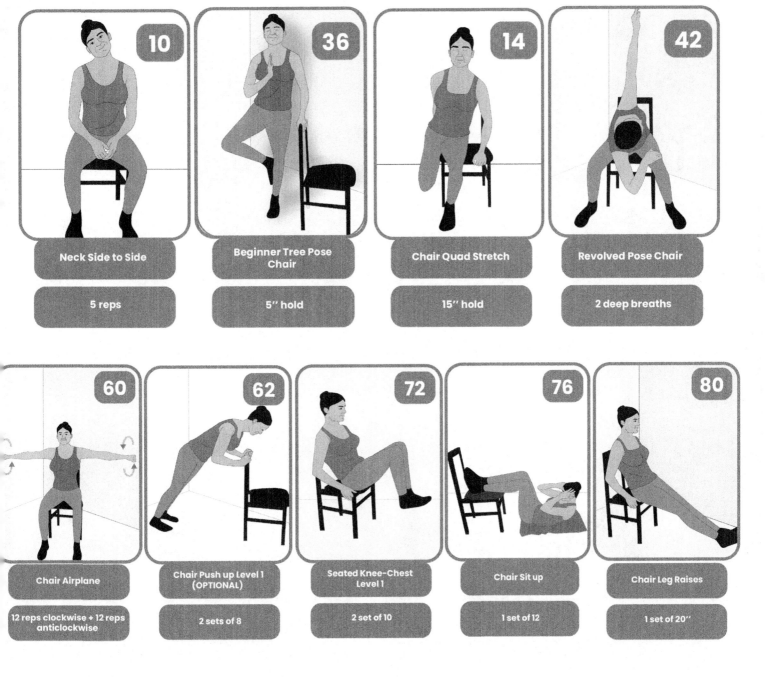

10 — Neck Side to Side — 5 reps

36 — Beginner Tree Pose Chair — 5″ hold

14 — Chair Quad Stretch — 15″ hold

42 — Revolved Pose Chair — 2 deep breaths

60 — Chair Airplane — 12 reps clockwise + 12 reps anticlockwise

62 — Chair Push up Level 1 (OPTIONAL) — 2 sets of 8

72 — Seated Knee-Chest Level 1 — 2 set of 10

76 — Chair Sit up — 1 set of 12

80 — Chair Leg Raises — 1 set of 20″

WEEK 02

WEDNESDAY

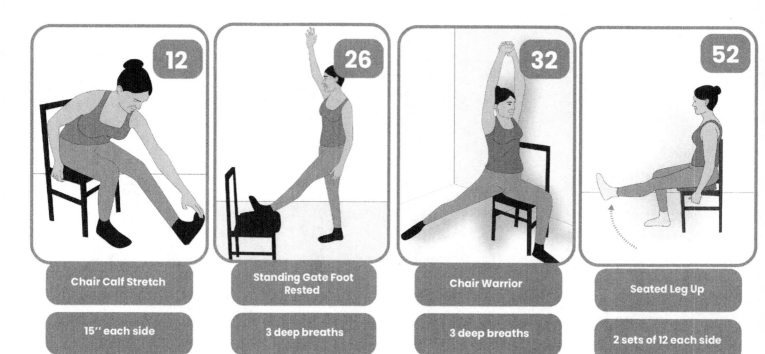

12 — Chair Calf Stretch — 15" each side

26 — Standing Gate Foot Rested — 3 deep breaths

32 — Chair Warrior — 3 deep breaths

52 — Seated Leg Up — 2 sets of 12 each side

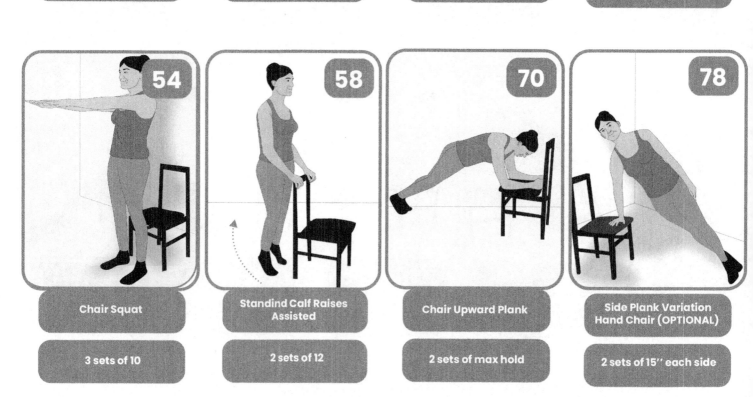

54 — Chair Squat — 3 sets of 10

58 — Standind Calf Raises Assisted — 2 sets of 12

70 — Chair Upward Plank — 2 sets of max hold

78 — Side Plank Variation Hand Chair (OPTIONAL) — 2 sets of 15" each side

WEEK 02

THURSDAY

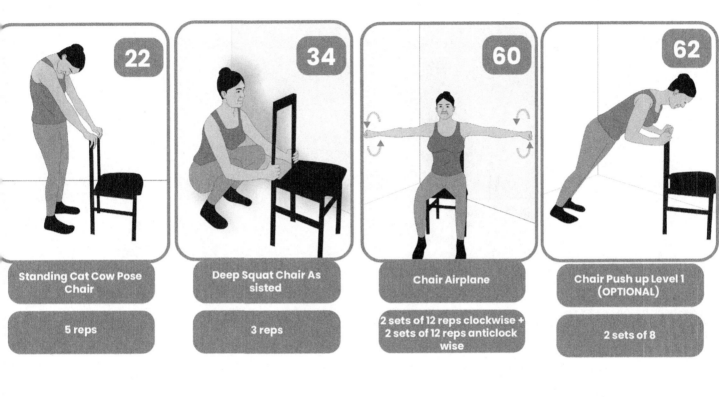

22
Standing Cat Cow Pose Chair

5 reps

34
Deep Squat Chair Assisted

3 reps

60
Chair Airplane

2 sets of 12 reps clockwise + 2 sets of 12 reps anticlock wise

62
Chair Push up Level 1 (OPTIONAL)

2 sets of 8

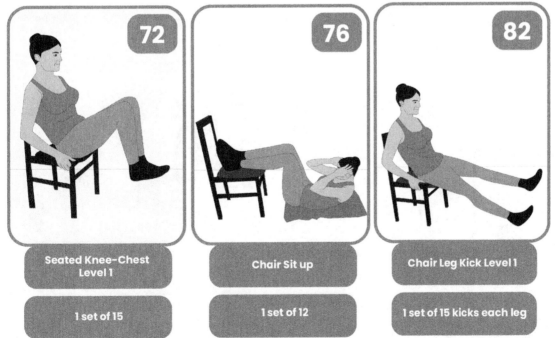

72
Seated Knee-Chest Level 1

1 set of 15

76
Chair Sit up

1 set of 12

82
Chair Leg Kick Level 1

1 set of 15 kicks each leg

WEEK 02

FRIDAY

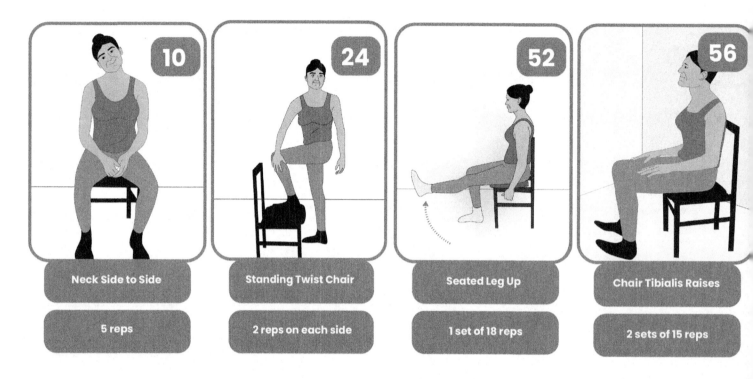

10

Neck Side to Side

5 reps

24

Standing Twist Chair

2 reps on each side

52

Seated Leg Up

1 set of 18 reps

56

Chair Tibialis Raises

2 sets of 15 reps

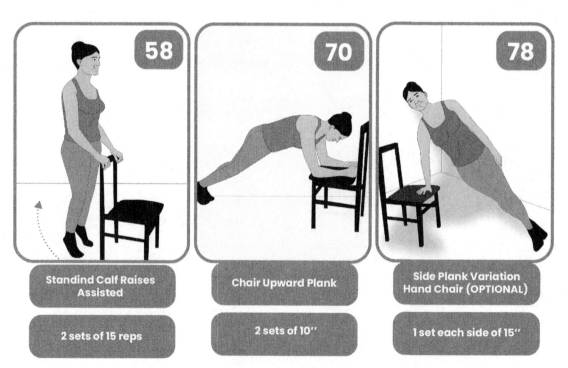

58

Standind Calf Raises Assisted

2 sets of 15 reps

70

Chair Upward Plank

2 sets of 10''

78

Side Plank Variation Hand Chair (OPTIONAL)

1 set each side of 15''

WEEK 02

SATURDAY

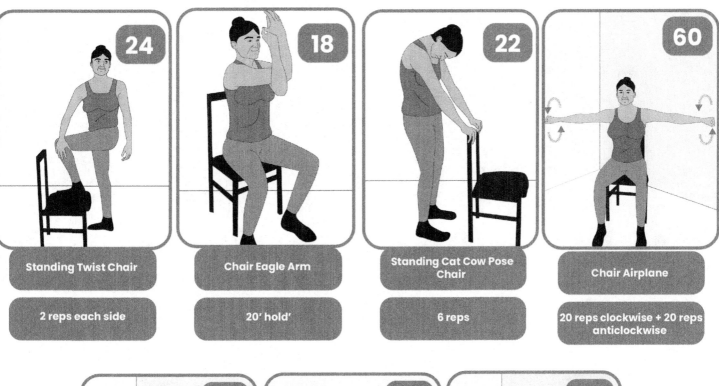

24	18	22	60
Standing Twist Chair	**Chair Eagle Arm**	**Standing Cat Cow Pose Chair**	**Chair Airplane**
2 reps each side	20' hold'	6 reps	20 reps clockwise + 20 reps anticlockwise

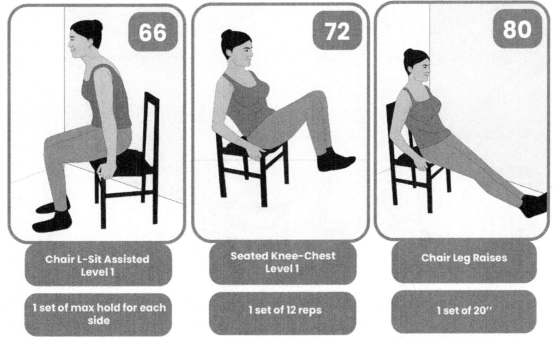

66	72	80
Chair L–Sit Assisted Level 1	**Seated Knee–Chest Level 1**	**Chair Leg Raises**
1 set of max hold for each side	1 set of 12 reps	1 set of 20''

SUNDAY: REST DAY

WEEK 03

MONDAY

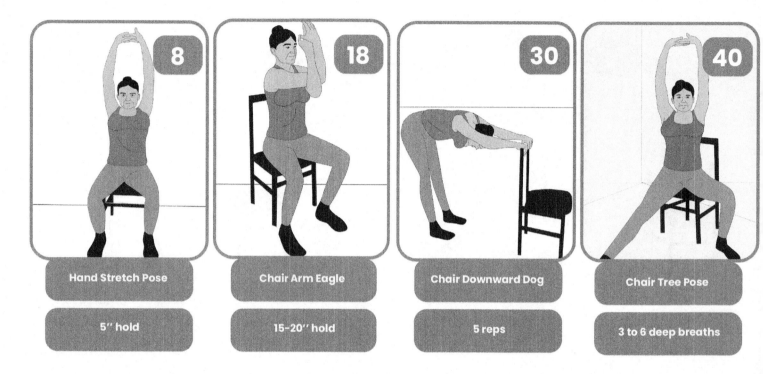

8 Hand Stretch Pose — 5" hold

18 Chair Arm Eagle — 15-20" hold

30 Chair Downward Dog — 5 reps

40 Chair Tree Pose — 3 to 6 deep breaths

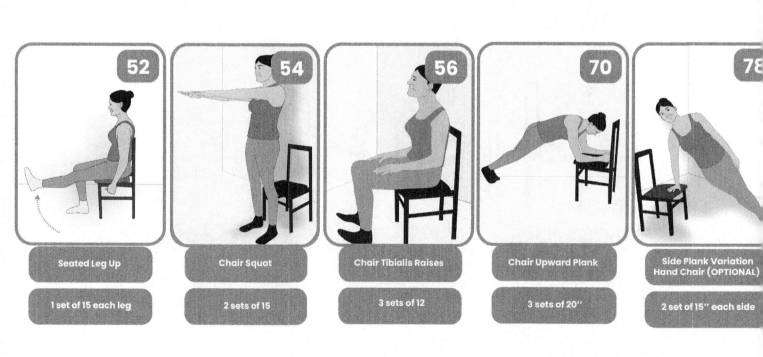

52 Seated Leg Up — 1 set of 15 each leg

54 Chair Squat — 2 sets of 15

56 Chair Tibialis Raises — 3 sets of 12

70 Chair Upward Plank — 3 sets of 20"

78 Side Plank Variation Hand Chair (OPTIONAL) — 2 set of 15" each side

WEEK 03

TUESDAY

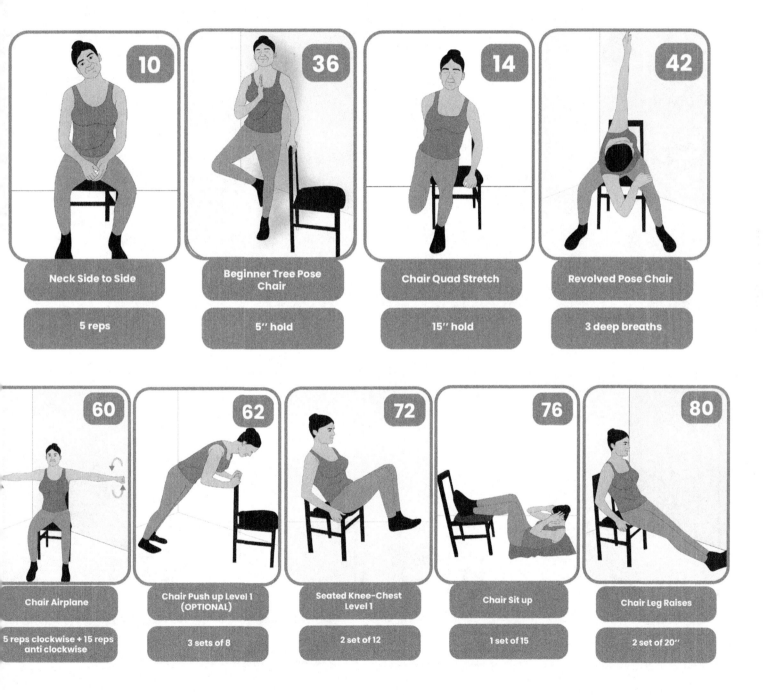

10
Neck Side to Side
5 reps

36
Beginner Tree Pose Chair
5'' hold

14
Chair Quad Stretch
15'' hold

42
Revolved Pose Chair
3 deep breaths

60
Chair Airplane
5 reps clockwise + 15 reps anti clockwise

62
Chair Push up Level 1 (OPTIONAL)
3 sets of 8

72
Seated Knee-Chest Level 1
2 set of 12

76
Chair Sit up
1 set of 15

80
Chair Leg Raises
2 set of 20''

WEEK 03

WEDNESDAY

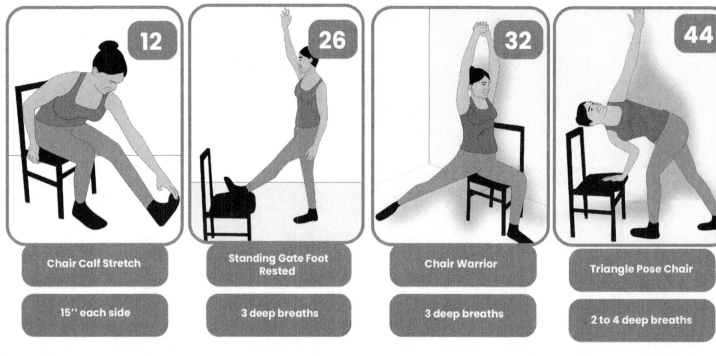

12 — Chair Calf Stretch
15'' each side

26 — Standing Gate Foot Rested
3 deep breaths

32 — Chair Warrior
3 deep breaths

44 — Triangle Pose Chair
2 to 4 deep breaths

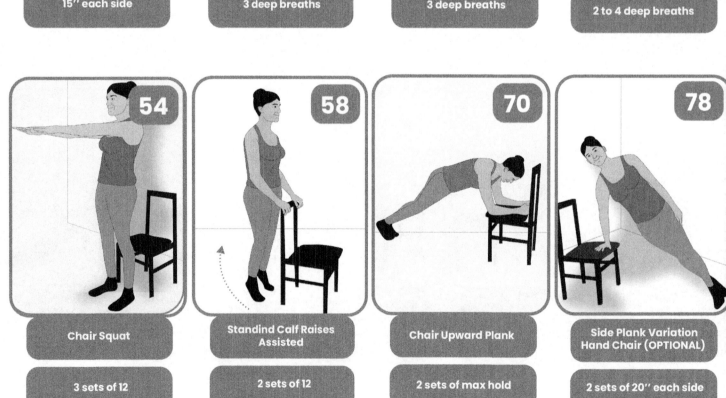

54 — Chair Squat
3 sets of 12

58 — Standind Calf Raises Assisted
2 sets of 12

70 — Chair Upward Plank
2 sets of max hold

78 — Side Plank Variation Hand Chair (OPTIONAL)
2 sets of 20'' each side

WEEK 03

THURSDAY

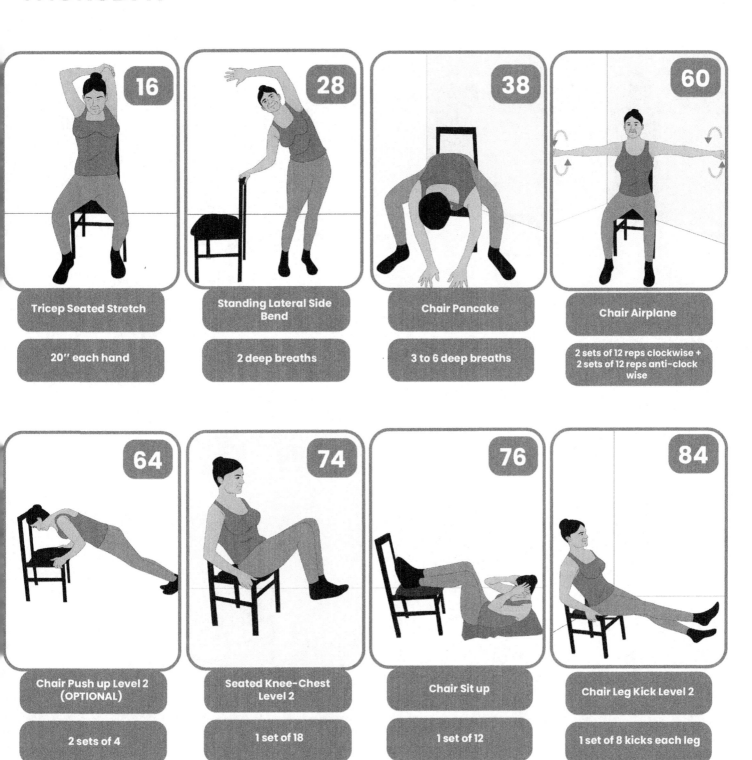

16
Tricep Seated Stretch

20'' each hand

28
Standing Lateral Side Bend

2 deep breaths

38
Chair Pancake

3 to 6 deep breaths

60
Chair Airplane

2 sets of 12 reps clockwise + 2 sets of 12 reps anti-clock wise

64
Chair Push up Level 2 (OPTIONAL)

2 sets of 4

74
Seated Knee-Chest Level 2

1 set of 18

76
Chair Sit up

1 set of 12

84
Chair Leg Kick Level 2

1 set of 8 kicks each leg

WEEK 03

FRIDAY

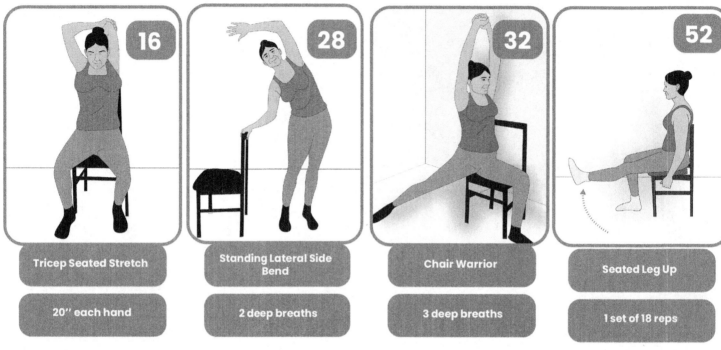

16 — Tricep Seated Stretch — 20" each hand

28 — Standing Lateral Side Bend — 2 deep breaths

32 — Chair Warrior — 3 deep breaths

52 — Seated Leg Up — 1 set of 18 reps

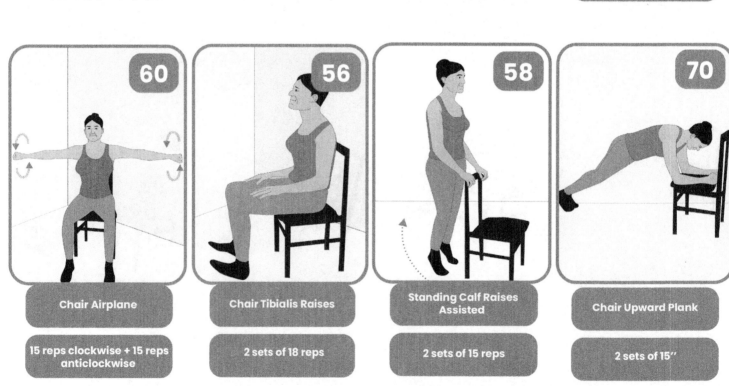

60 — Chair Airplane — 15 reps clockwise + 15 reps anticlockwise

56 — Chair Tibialis Raises — 2 sets of 18 reps

58 — Standing Calf Raises Assisted — 2 sets of 15 reps

70 — Chair Upward Plank — 2 sets of 15"

WEEK 03

SATURDAY

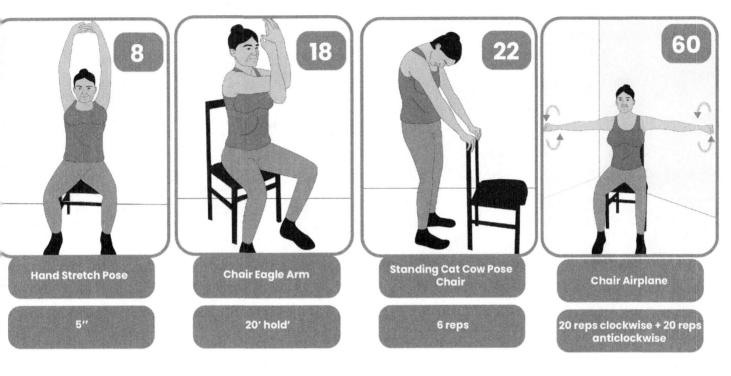

Hand Stretch Pose	**Chair Eagle Arm**	**Standing Cat Cow Pose Chair**	**Chair Airplane**
5''	20' hold'	6 reps	20 reps clockwise + 20 reps anticlockwise

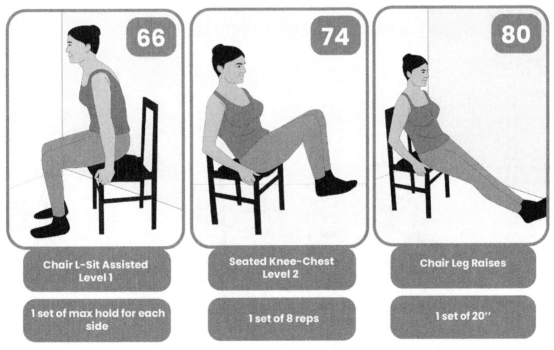

Chair L-Sit Assisted Level 1	**Seated Knee-Chest Level 2**	**Chair Leg Raises**
1 set of max hold for each side	1 set of 8 reps	1 set of 20''

SUNDAY: REST DAY

WEEK 04

MONDAY

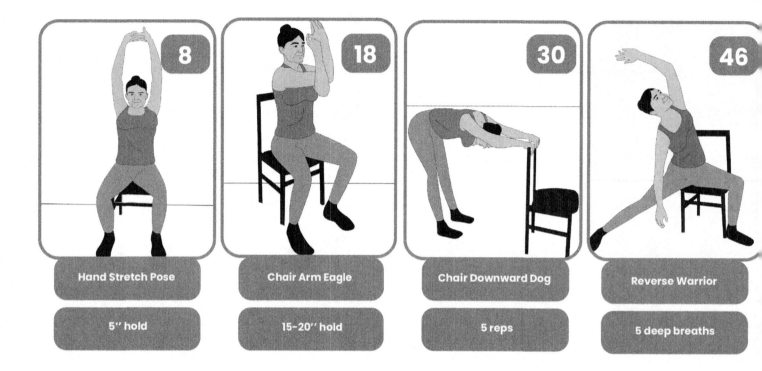

Hand Stretch Pose

5'' hold

Chair Arm Eagle

15-20'' hold

Chair Downward Dog

5 reps

Reverse Warrior

5 deep breaths

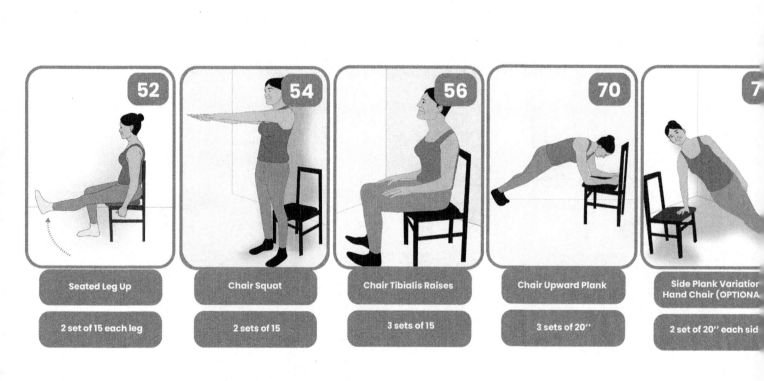

Seated Leg Up

2 set of 15 each leg

Chair Squat

2 sets of 15

Chair Tibialis Raises

3 sets of 15

Chair Upward Plank

3 sets of 20''

Side Plank Variation Hand Chair (OPTIONAL

2 set of 20'' each sid

TUESDAY

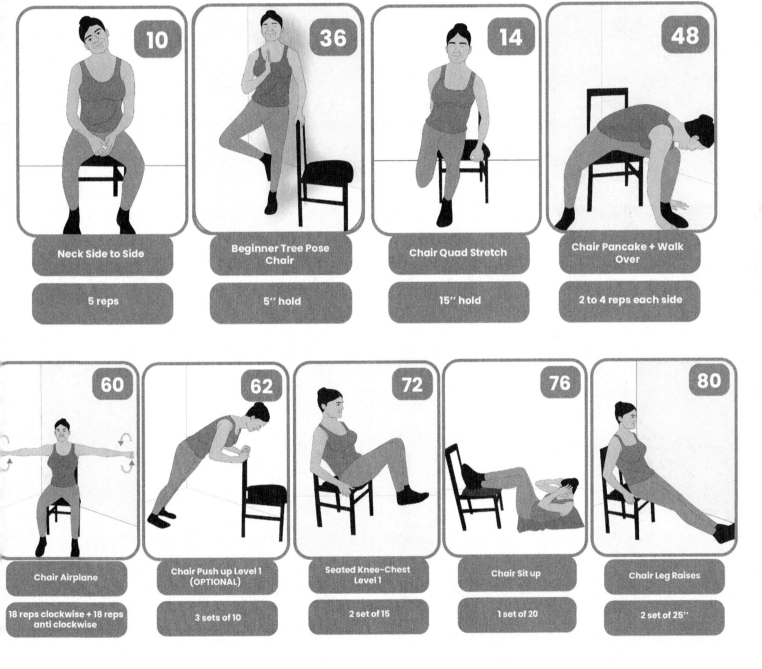

10 Neck Side to Side — 5 reps

36 Beginner Tree Pose Chair — 5" hold

14 Chair Quad Stretch — 15" hold

48 Chair Pancake + Walk Over — 2 to 4 reps each side

60 Chair Airplane — 18 reps clockwise + 18 reps anti clockwise

62 Chair Push up Level 1 (OPTIONAL) — 3 sets of 10

72 Seated Knee-Chest Level 1 — 2 set of 15

76 Chair Sit up — 1 set of 20

80 Chair Leg Raises — 2 set of 25"

WEDNESDAY

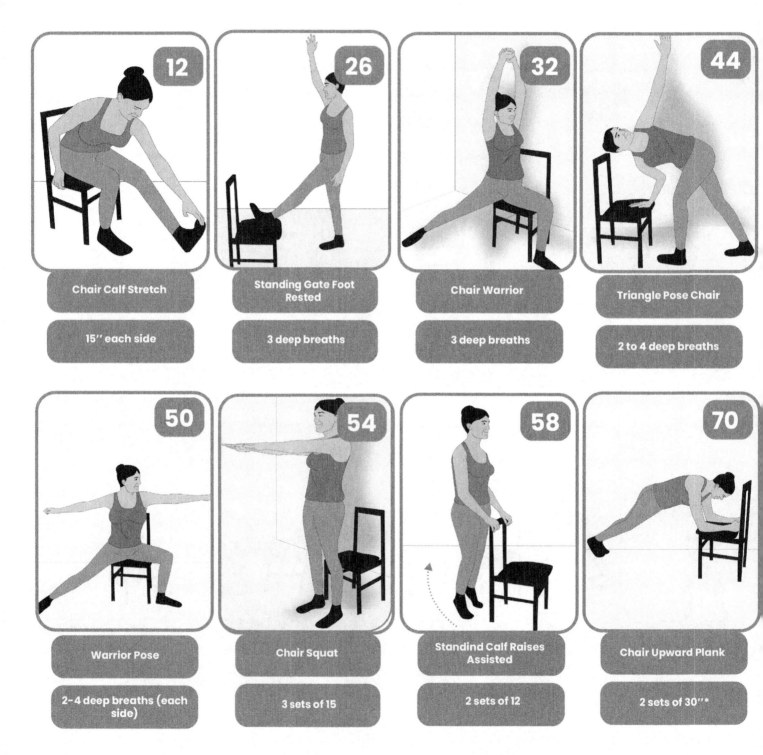

12
Chair Calf Stretch
15'' each side

26
Standing Gate Foot Rested
3 deep breaths

32
Chair Warrior
3 deep breaths

44
Triangle Pose Chair
2 to 4 deep breaths

50
Warrior Pose
2–4 deep breaths (each side)

54
Chair Squat
3 sets of 15

58
Standind Calf Raises Assisted
2 sets of 12

70
Chair Upward Plank
2 sets of 30''*

*30'' IS THE GOAL. IF YOU STILL CANNOT DO IT, NO PROBLEM, JUST DO YOUR BEST!

WEEK 04

THURSDAY

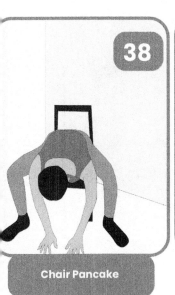

38

Chair Pancake

3 to 6 deep breaths

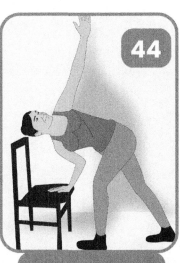

44

Triangle Pose Chair

4 deep breaths

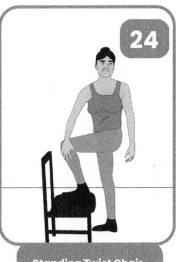

24

Standing Twist Chair

2 reps each side (3 deep breaths on each rep)

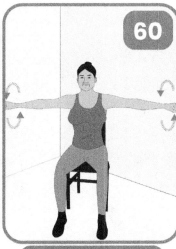

60

Chair Airplane

2 sets of 15 reps clockwise + 2 sets of 15 reps anti-clock wise

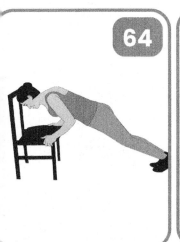

64

Chair Push up Level 2 (OPTIONAL)

2 sets of 48

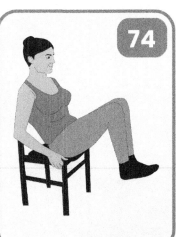

74

Seated Knee-Chest Level 2

1 set of 12

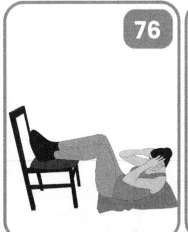

76

Chair Sit up

1 set of 15

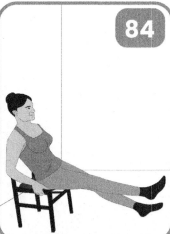

84

Chair Leg Kick Level 2

1 set of 10 kicks each leg

FRIDAY

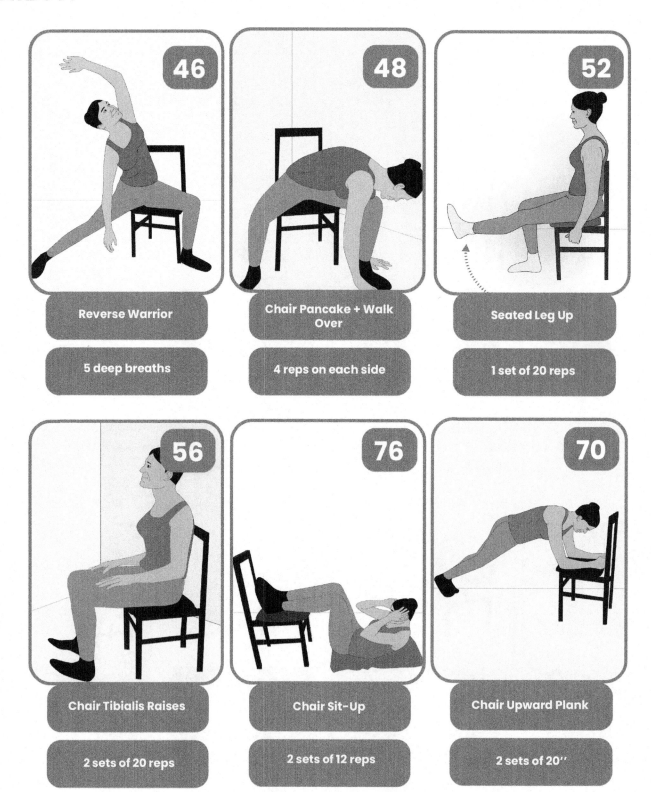

46

Reverse Warrior

5 deep breaths

48

Chair Pancake + Walk Over

4 reps on each side

52

Seated Leg Up

1 set of 20 reps

56

Chair Tibialis Raises

2 sets of 20 reps

76

Chair Sit-Up

2 sets of 12 reps

70

Chair Upward Plank

2 sets of 20''

WEEK 04

SATURDAY

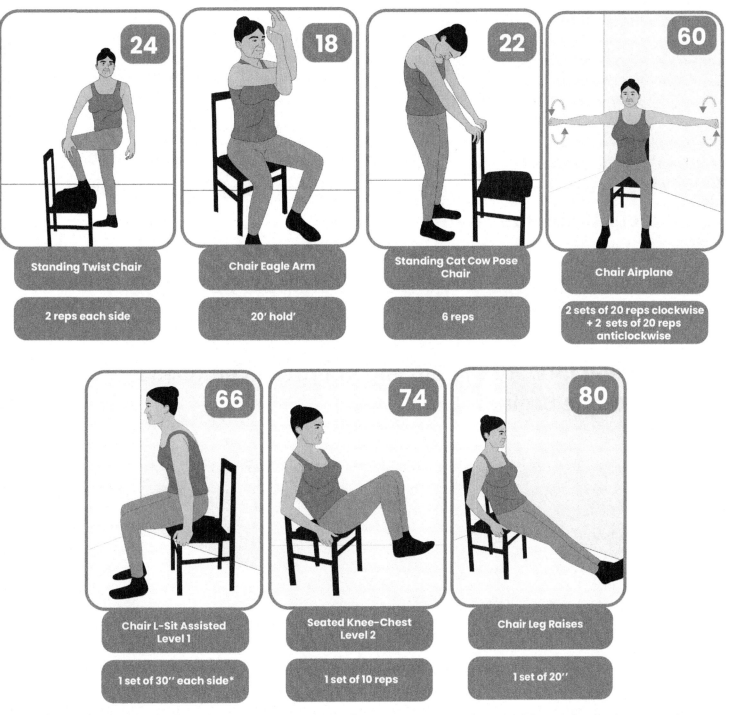

24 — Standing Twist Chair — 2 reps each side

18 — Chair Eagle Arm — 20' hold'

22 — Standing Cat Cow Pose Chair — 6 reps

60 — Chair Airplane — 2 sets of 20 reps clockwise + 2 sets of 20 reps anticlockwise

66 — Chair L-Sit Assisted Level 1 — 1 set of 30'' each side*

74 — Seated Knee-Chest Level 2 — 1 set of 10 reps

80 — Chair Leg Raises — 1 set of 20''

*30'' is the goal for this 4-week plan. If you cannot, no problem, just do your best!

SUNDAY: REST DAY

Have you finished the 4-Week plan and are you looking to continue your training?

Contact me at avfitness99coaching@gmail.com or visit my Instagram profile - avfitness99

Looking forward to help you improve even further...this is just the beginning!

HEALTHY LIFESTYLE TIPS THAT WILL 10X YOUR FITNESS RESULTS

I am sure that by following the 30-Day Challenge you will feel 10x better. What's next?

You can definitely keep improving in the exercises and get more results. However, exercise is just a small part of your day. Creating good habits is key for living well and for long! Here are some key tips.

- **Go outside in the morning**

Regardless if it's sunny, rainy, or cloudy, going outside for anywhere between 10 and 30 minutes after waking up is crucial for optimizing your well-being.

Many studies have been done on the importance and impact on sunlight, especially early in the morning as it helps falling asleep way faster, also improving sleep's quality. It also has an impact on many other things, such as:

▸ Mood and emotional well-being.

▸ Production of melatonin, then released at night.

▸ Hormones regulation and increased level of dopamine during the day.

▸ Ability to Focus more and for longer.

▸ Immune function boost.

- **Avoid blue lights before going to sleep.**

Sleep is extremely important for your well-being and for your fitness. Screen time decrease melatonin release so that makes more difficult and less effective our sleep and recovery. Making sure that the quality of it is as high as possible is crucial (especially if you cannot sleep 8/9 hours at night).

Also, going to sleep at the same time every day will improve your hormonal health making you more energized during the day.

Note: In general, a good guide to have is to spend more time outside during the day and less screen time, especially the first hours after waking up, and before going to sleep. Simple rule that gives amazing results in terms of health, productivity, and well-being!

- **Eat mindfully.**

It does not matter only what you eat; if you eat too much food, you will be tired. Ideally, you will not go above 85% of fullness to avoid that feeling.

Also, drink more water throughout the day and prioritize healthy food not processed too much as it will be difficult to digest and most likely, not giving you the right macronutrients, your body needs to perform at its best!

- **Meditate 10 minutes a day.**

This is a practice that can be done anywhere. It might be easier if you find a slot during the day to keep it as a habit (as soon as you wake up or before going to sleep are exceptionally good options). You will definitely feel more centered, calm in stressful situations and in control of your actions if you stick with it for a few weeks.

 If you have tried meditation, but you do not think it is highly effective for you, try NSDR. It's a guided relaxation technique that helps tremendously! YouTube has a lot of videos about it that you can watch.

- **Decrease drastically, or avoid completely, alcoholic drinks.**

Many scientific studies proved that there are no benefits in alcohol consumption. Several studies have shown that even modest consumption of alcohol can lead to people becoming more stressed and less resilient eventually. It also has an impact on depression, obesity, and overall low level of energy.

"Alcohol is the only drug where if you don't do it, people assume you have a problem." Cit. Chris Williamson

CONCLUSION

This guide comes to an end!

If you started reading this book because you felt frail, with fear of falling and/or with limited mobility, I am 100% sure that this illustrated guide helped you immensely!

At times I am sure, as it is normal, that you will experience difficulties and struggles during the workouts.

That's part of the process. If you stick with it for 28-days following the indications and the step-by-step instructions, on the other side there's a more independent life that will make you feel physically active once again!

Thanks a lot for reading the book!

ABOUT ME

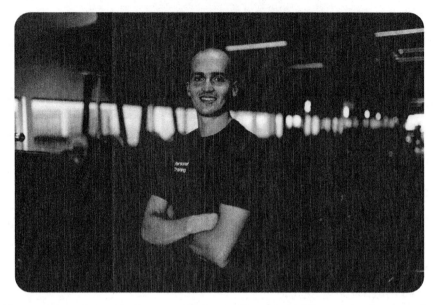

My name is Alessandro, I am Italian, and I have lived in Milan, London, and now Valencia, Spain. My passion for fitness started in my childhood and never stopped since then.

I am a certified Personal Trainer with years of experience in the United Kingdom and Spain. I have been studying fitness articles and guides to make people fitter for years. My experience helping hundreds of people led me to write numerous books on it.

The goal is to make them healthier, more flexible, stronger, and enjoy life more.

I have been doing 1-on-1 sessions, group sessions and online coaching with people of all ages. However, I gained more experience in the last few years with people over 50 and 60. Hence why my passion in helping them skyrocketed, leasing to write a guide to get to as many people as possible.

I dream of a world in which age is just a number!

I published many books to help seniors living their best life! My source of motivation started from my childhood. I loved spending time with my grandad in the garden, and I always wished we could play for hours. However, that was not possible as he could not endure too much physical exercise. With years, seeing some physical problems that he was enduring made me willing to help him, even though as a teenager, I did not have any information and knowledge to practically help you. After more than a decade, I want to make grandparents play with their nephews and nieces for hours without stopping for lack of strength, balance, flexibility or because they are tired.

This is my mission, and I hope to reach it with these simple guides!

💪Other Books Available for you on Amazon💪

1. **Wall Pilates for Seniors: Rediscover The Joy of Movement and Become Independent Once Again with Low-Impact Exercises to Improve Flexibility and Balance**

Fantastic to approach Wall Pilates exercises with low-impact exercises in just 10-15 minutes per day - Plan of 30 days included.

2. **Wall Pilates Workouts: 28-Day Challenge with Exercise Chart for Weight Loss | 10-Min Routines for Women, Beginners and Seniors - Color Illustrated Edition**

The newest book! Fully colored, Video tutorials, graphic routines and downloadable exercise charts ... .the best to lose weight and burn fat at home!

3. **Chair Yoga for Seniors: 28-Day Challenge for Weight Loss with Exercise Chart | 10-Min Low-Impact Routines for Beginners - Color Illustrated Edition**

Color illustrated, easy-to-follow, step-by-step illustrations, printable exercise charts and direct access to text me anytime you need...

4. **Chair Yoga for Weight Loss: 28-Day Challenge to Lose Belly Fat Sitting Downwith Low-Impact Exercises in Just 10 Minutes Per Day**

Arguably the best book to burn calories, lose weight and improve flexibility with low-impact daily routines!

5. **Balance Exercises Bible for Seniors: 12-Week Plan to Prevent Falls and Walking with Confidence in Under 10 Minutes a Day | Pictures Included for Easy Understanding**

Plenty of exercises to choose from for beginners, intermediate and advanced - 12-week plan and so much more!

Scan the QR Code to Go to My Amazon Profile and Get the Book you Prefer

QR Code for USA

QR Code for UK

QR Code for Canada

Printed in Great Britain
by Amazon

46727789R00073